A HISTORY OF THE COUNCIL FOR THE EDUCATION AND TRAINING OF HEALTH VISITORS

THE MIDDLE YEARS

Published by the Council for the Education and Training of Health Visitors.

The Work of the Nursing Team in General Practice.

An Investigation into the Principles of Health Visiting.

The Investigation Debate.

Health Visiting Principles in Practice

The History of the Council for the Education and Training of Health Visitors.

Teaching for Reality.

An Evaluation of Health Visiting.

First published in 1983

ISBN: 0 946810 00 1

Printed by Duncan Printing Co Ltd, Aylesford, Maidstone, Kent.

A History of the Council for the Education and Training of Health Visitors

An Account of its Activities 1975-1980

NORMA BATLEY

English National Board for Nursing, Midwifery
and Health Visiting

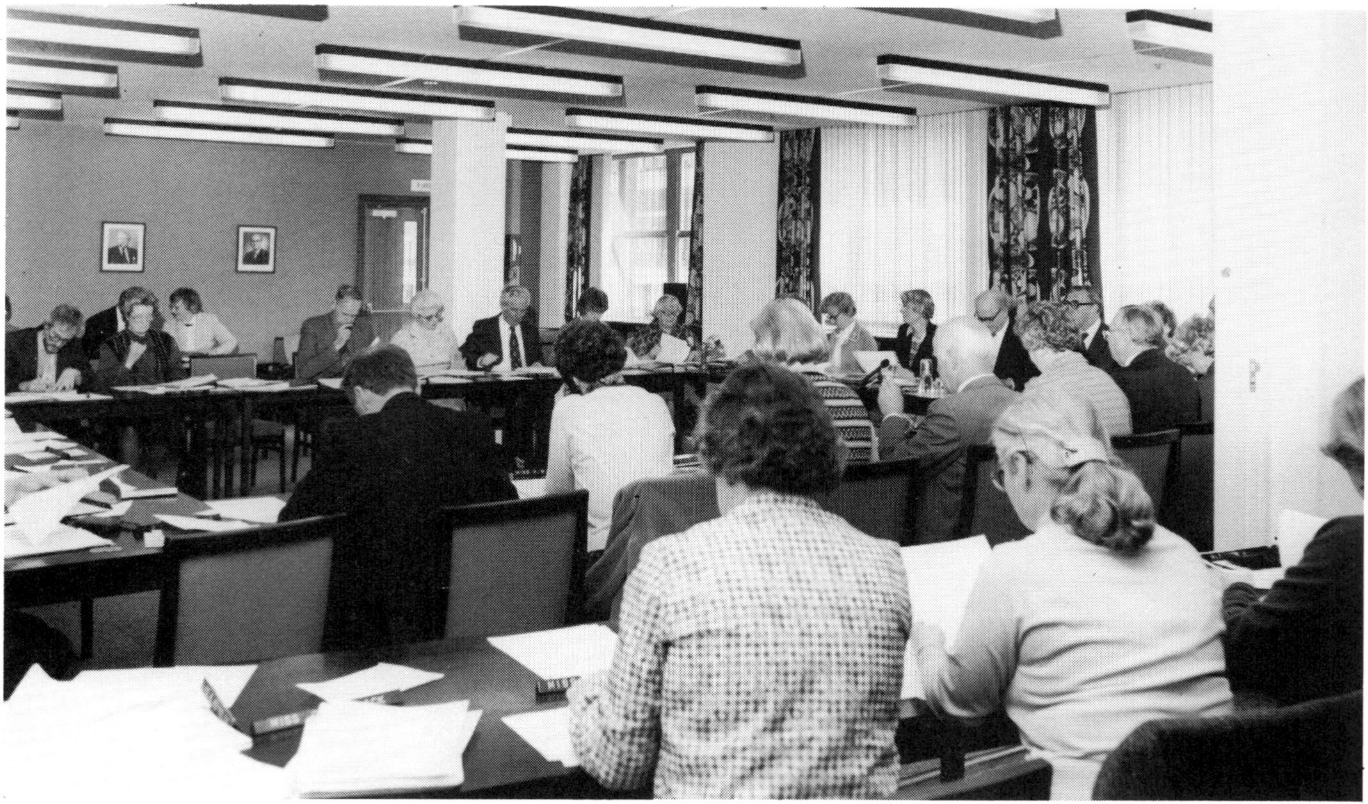

The 7th Council in Session

Introduction by the Chairman of the Council for the Education and Training of Health Visitors

This book is a sequel to 'The History of the Council for the Education and Training of Health Visitors' which was written by the first Director, Miss Elaine Wilkie and published in 1979. Miss Wilkie's book deals with the period from the establishment of the Council in 1962 until its separation from the Central Council for the Education and Training in Social Work in 1975. It was thus concerned with the establishment of courses in higher and further education, the very large expansion of student numbers, the introduction of the new syllabus and the development of courses for health visitor tutors and fieldwork teachers.

In contrast, the period covered by this book has been one of relative stability of student numbers and the consolidation of courses in higher and further education. Nevertheless, important new developments have occurred, including the extension of the fieldwork teacher course to two years and the provision of a Council Certificate for those who successfully complete it; the development of courses for assessors of supervised practice; the examination of the whole field of continuing education for health visitors and the establishment of a category of recognised courses of continuing education; and further detailed consideration of the curriculum of the health visitors course. A further innovation has been the development of courses in school nursing. Perhaps the most important events of this period, however, have been those connected with and leading up to the implementation of the Nurses, Midwives and Health Visitors Act 1979.

The Council was very much concerned to ensure that what had been achieved for health visitor education and training should continue under the new Act. The Director during 'The Middle Years', Miss Norma Batley exhibited great persistence and dedication to the cause of health visitor education and training during the complex and protracted negotiations which accompanied the passage of the Bill through Parliament. That part of the book, therefore, which provides Miss Batley's personal account of the negotiations and enables the reader to see, through her eyes, the intricacies and nuances of these negotiations is a valuable contribution to the history of health visitor education and training.

This book is a lucid, interesting and illuminating account of the mature years of an important statutory body and of its relationships with other similar organisations and with government at a time of profound change in the arrangements for the education, training and registration of nurses, midwives and health visitors.

CLIFFORD BUTLER

Abbreviations

ANO	Area Nursing Officer.
Briggs Report	Report of the Committee on Nursing. Chairman Professor Asa Briggs.
CANO	Chief Administrative Nursing Officer (Northern Ireland)/Chief Area Nursing Officer (Scotland)
CCETSW	Central Council for Education and Training in Social Work.
CETHV or "The Council"	Council for the Education and Training of Health Visitors.
EEC	European Economic Community.
DHSS	Department of Health and Society Security.
HV	Health Visitor.
HVA	Health Visitors' Association.
HVT	Health Visitor Tutor.
JBCNS	Joint Board of Clinical Nursing Studies.
NICNM	Northern Ireland Council for Nurses and Midwives.
RCN	Royal College of Nursing.
RNO	Regional Nursing Officer.
SHHD	Scottish Home and Health Department.
The 1962 Act	Health Visiting and Social Work (Training) Act 1962.
The 1979 Act	Nurses, Midwives and Health Visitors Act 1979.

Foreword

This book is dedicated to the members of Council and the members of staff past and present with whom I worked with so much pleasure and who by giving unstintingly of their time and skill were responsible for the continuing development of the work of the Council for the Education and Training of Health Visitors from 1975-80. Particular thanks are offered to all who were concerned in the preparation of this book before it reached the printers. I should like especially to mention two members of the Council for the Education and Training of Health Visitors, Margaret Illing and Professor Ian Richardson, who gave guidance as readers of the manuscript in draft; and Margaret Thwaites the Director, Pamela Hay, Henry Turner, Richard Stanwell and the patient secretarial staff for their constant encouragement and help.

The "History of the Council for the Education and Training of Health Visitors" by Elaine Wilkie contained a resumé of events leading up to the establishment of the CTHV (later CETHV) following the Health Visiting and Social Work (Training) Act of 1962, of the ways in which the Council set about its tasks and of all that was accomplished in the first twelve years, 1962-1975. The purpose of this second book is to place on record the work of the Council during the subsequent period from 1975-1980, which might be described as "The Middle Years", between the 'foundation' period already recorded and the final phase of its life during which it will be involved in the handover of its functions to the Central Council, National Boards and the Health Visiting Joint Committee, as the Nurses, Midwives and Health Visitors Act of 1979 is implemented.

In these circumstances, an attempt has been made to link this account of the work in the 'Middle Years' with that contained in "The History of the CETHV" and to include reference to some of the reasoning which lay behind the actions taken. At the same time, because of the pending changes, particular reference has been made to the Council's methods of work and its experience as a U.K. Statutory Body - one of a number of pioneering roles of the CETHV during its comparatively short but very active life.

Although business arising out of the preparations for the Nurses, Midwives and Health Visitors Act continued throughout this 5 year period, making exceptional demands upon members and staff alike, a factual account of these events is left to the final section only so as to leave intact the record of the Council as it developed the statutory functions prescribed for it under the terms of the 1962 Act.

In Section 5, "The Passage of the Nurses, Midwives and Health Visitors Bill 1979" no attempt has been made to describe the total situation as it developed. What I have attempted is to describe, mainly in the form of quotations from relevant documents of the time, events of particular significance to the Council, which best display the consistent policy it pursued and the reasons for the various actions taken.

If the "Summary" appears disproportionately long, this is because the aim has been to offer reasonably comprehensive notes for the interest of those in full-time employment who have little opportunity to digest the volume of reading material that comes their way. And finally, the "Postscript by the Author" contains personal and genuinely held views in contrast with the factually based material elsewhere and for these I take full responsibility.

Supplements to the Sections have been interspersed throughout. Some are in their original form and are no more than 'working papers'. Nevertheless, it is hoped they will serve to illustrate further the business carried out by the Council during the 'Middle Years', the years in which the Council first attained its own separate staff and premises and before it entered the final phase of its life as a fully independent Statutory Body.

N.B.B.
Spring 1982

Apologies must be offered now to the Council that due to adverse circumstances publication has been delayed for a year. Also particular thanks must be recorded to Dr Henry Turner who took on the onerous additional task of editing the script.

N.B.B.
Spring 1983

Contents

106

SECTION 1

THE MIDDLE YEARS

The first nationally recognised examinations leading to the award of Health Visitor Certificates were organised by the Royal Sanitary Institutes of England and of Scotland respectively in the 1920s. Arrangements for these examinations were modified over the years and were finally terminated with the implementation of the Health Visiting and Social Work (Training) Act 1962. This Act, which led to the establishment of the Council for the Training of Health Visitors (later the Council for the Education and Training of Health Visitors) gave wide statutory powers to this Council for the approval of courses for Health Visitors, recruitment, further education, the provision of examinations and for research, and applied to the whole of the United Kingdom. "The History of the Council for the Education and Training of Health Visitors" by Elaine Wilkie recorded the first 12 years of the Council's life and displayed the twofold influences on the development of its work - the effects of external events and of the initiatives taken by the Council itself.

In Section 1 of this second "History", this general theme is carried forward to cover the years 1975 - 1980 and continues to emphasise both the complementary and the conflicting effects of these two influences.

Developments within the Health and Education Services and their effect on the work of the Council

If "no man is an island", then by the same token the Council cannot function effectively without being acutely aware of and influenced by external events. During the "Middle Years", these influences have been substantial; and some have been encouraging and some disturbing.

In the first place, the Council had every reason to feel encouraged by those publications from both Government and other sources which appeared to indicate a new awakening of interest in prevention and to stress the importance of the contributions that might be made by Health Visitors (see Section 1 Supplement 1). Together with this, the initiative taken by the Council in establishing courses for Health Visitors in institutions of Higher and Further Education was by now proving its worth and the Council was beginning to gain the benefits of innovations arising from the work of the staff, and from the policies, of these educational establishments; the Health Visitors

Tutors had gained from the experience of working with lecturers in many other disciplines and the Health Visitor students were expressing appreciation of this wider form of education.

Other developments, however, gave cause for concern. While the merits and demerits of the Reorganisation of the National Health Service in 1974 will be argued elsewhere, as far as the work of the Council was concerned it caused major disruptions and the practical problems which it caused were considerable. No longer was there to be a 'pooling' system to finance Health Visitor students, no longer was there to be a Chief Officer within the Local Health Authority directly responsible for and knowledgeable about Health Visiting with whom the Council could communicate, no longer was there to be a management structure in Health Visiting per se and no longer was it certain that newly qualified Health Visitors would have the essential support from Nursing Officers/Health Visitors which was necessary if they were to become competent practitioners. Authorities were being established in some places without Community Divisions and it became difficult for the Council to remain informed about service policies and practices in the Health Visitor's work-place of Primary Care.

The immediate result of these changes was the need for a massive "public relations exercise" to inform those Nursing Managers who were unfamiliar with the work of the Council and in many cases with the practices of the institutions of Higher and Further Education, of the responsibilities of this Statutory Body and also to encourage them to recruit and fund Health Visitor students. In practical terms, this required visits to be made by the Council's Professional Advisers to all parts of the U.K. and discussion to be held with literally hundreds of Managers, either individually or in groups. The institutions of Higher and Further Education too were faced with the problem of communicating with Service Managers, who were still uncertain of their own role, about such matters as student selection and the provision of practical work. The problems of corresponding with several levels of management, which had been the cause of complaint in particular in the English schools (where it was found in one case the arrangements for placing a student had needed 30 letters), was brought to the attention of the DHSS and was partially resolved by a letter to Nursing Officers from the Chief Nursing Officer which advised that enquiries should be channelled through one member of staff (Ref 1). The decline in student numbers that followed Reorganisation was the subject of investigations carried out by the Council which revealed a number of different causes. All in all, however, the very serious fact remained that recruitment never recovered from the effects of the Reorganisation of the National Health Service in 1974 (see Appendix

(Ref 1) CNO 75/8 - Health Visitor Training

2), the downward trend contrasting sharply with the substantial increases which had been recorded in earlier years.

A number of other events also caused the Council deep concern. The Halsbury Report which led to the rationalisation of salaries for the whole nursing profession eliminated the salary differentials as between Health Visitors and Fieldwork Teachers. This lack of recognition of the responsibility of the Fieldwork Teacher in financial terms was a continuing cause of complaint throughout the 'Middle Years' and led to the threat of disruption in arrangements for Health Visitor students' practical work. The policy of the Council in insisting on a system of training for those in charge of the students' practical work have been an exceptional advance which had been commented on favourably by some of H.M. Inspectors of Schools familiar with a wide range of courses for the professions.

It was therefore particularly disquieting that these Health Visitors, who had undertaken further training in order to provide a more skilled service to the students in the practical aspects of Health Visiting, should be disadvantaged by the change in the salary structure. The Council continued to make representations to the Whitley Council for the removal of this anomaly and expressed its gratitude to the Fieldwork Teachers for their continued loyalty to the profession and to the interests of the students.

The EEC Directives for Midwives and for Nurses, which again were matters totally outside the influence of the Council, posed considerable problems. In respect of midwifery, it became evident that the likely changes in midwifery courses and in the arrangements for midwifery experience to be acquired for student nurses would disrupt the established pattern of course recognised by the Council in order to meet the statutory requirement in midwifery or obstetrics for intending Health Visitor students. It became necessary therefore to enter into negotiations first with the CMB (Scotland), subsequently with the NICNM and finally with the CMB (England and Wales) in order to plan and eventually to implement new courses in obstetrics. These new courses were based on syllabuses designed by the CETHV in co-operation with the appropriate Statutory Bodies for Midwifery taking account of the advice of Midwife Teachers and Health Visitor Tutors. Early reports suggested that the students were finding the specially designed courses helpful. The whole exercise, which was very demanding in time and energy for all concerned, exemplified the co-operation already enjoyed through the constructive relationships which had been established with other Statutory Bodies. The problem of finance, however, remained. While, as had happened in the past, intending Health Visitor students attended courses arranged primarily for Midwives or for Student Nurses the cost was insignificant. The establishment of separate courses, however, meant that considerable sums of extra money were now needed to finance the attendance of an increasing number of students. This potential problem was brought to the attention of the DHSS in advance of the signing of the relevant Directives but remained unresolved. Service Managers, faced with the problem of meeting from their budgets the demands both for financing the service and for the training of staff, sometimes felt that they were unable to meet this additional expense. Meanwhile, it was known that potential recruits for Health Visiting courses were being lost because individuals found themselves unable to gain the necessary prerequisite qualifications in obstetrics.

The establishment of a specially designed obstetric course for intending Health Visitor students suggested the possibility similarly of devising a special course in nursing for those who wished to qualify as Health Visitors and had no particular wish to take the full training to become a Registered Nurse. While this question has been discussed informally on a number of occasions, there was no pressure on the Council during this period to undertake the extensive investigations that would have been necessary before any such radical change could be contemplated. Furthermore, action of this nature would have been ill-timed while the negotiations regarding the 1979 Act were in progress even if it had been otherwise considered desirable.

Apart from the issue of obstetric courses, the EEC Directives for Nursing did not pose any immediate problems to those engaged in Health Visitor Education and Training, except by increasing the demand by student nurses for experience with practising Health Visitors, who might already be engaged as Fieldwork Teachers in teaching Health Visitor students. However, it was particularly helpful to the Council that the working group of the Council's Scottish Advisory Committee took part in discussions with the GNC (Scotland) on the content of the proposed "Community Module" in its new GNC syllabus and gave some consideration to the effect this might have on the Health Visitor course. In Northern Ireland too, the Advisory Committee had the benefit of a talk on the developments in nursing education from a representative of the Northern Ireland Council for Nurses and Midwives.

The most serious problems in the provision of Health Visitor education and training in 'Middle Years' arose from events outside the control of or, it appears, the influence of the Council. This suggests that unless the secondary effects on Health Visitors of radical changes made in the interests of large groups of nurses are appreciated and provision made for the safe-guarding of the interests of such a minority group, accommodating the interests of the larger group may act - and in some instances has acted - directly to the detriment of the smaller. Furthermore, in the absence of an appreciation of the 'knock-on' effects of such changes and the provision of safeguards, damage was caused and situations had to be retrieved, as far as possible, with much difficulty and at great cost in terms of human time and energy. The dilemma facing the Council therefore remained: although the Government had asked for a new initiative in Preventive and Community Services and the Council and some employing authorities were doing their best to respond, significant decision making elsewhere appeared to remain focused on arrangements for the larger number of Hospital Nurses. From the view point of the Council, it appeared that no action was taken in response to the Government's intention to expand the development of Health Visiting but rather the reverse - as is illustrated above.

With responsibilities extending throughout the U.K., the Council has had to be aware of the policies of all U.K. Health Departments and also of the U.K. Education Departments. In 1976, the issue of the "grading of courses" in Colleges i.e. the criteria employed in the Public Sector of Education to describe the level of a course, came under scrutiny and the Council made representations in respect of the Health Visitor courses to the Burnham Committee in England and the Ferguson Committee in Scotland as their decisions might have had significance in relation to the staffing of Health Visitor courses.

The final decisions by these Committees graded the Health Visitor course as Category II/III in England and as Grade II in Scotland. This was an example of the differences sometimes encountered 'north and south of the border', differences which had to be respected and which, while they generated extra work, did not necessarily cause difficulties. Arrangements for the provision of Health Visitor courses in institutions of Higher and Further Education on the whole worked smoothly by now and cases of major difficulties arising between the Council and the Education Institutions or Authorities were very rare. In keeping with the mood of the times, however, it was felt to be prudent to prepare documents setting out the precise responsibilities of both the Council on the one hand and the institutions on the other to cover, for example, the situation which might arise should students dispute their examination results.

The Council's decision to establish Health Visitor education and training in institutions of Higher and Further Education had proved timely (Ref 2). In a period of growth and development, it had been possible to ensure that on the one hand the statutory responsibilities of the Council and, on the other, compliance with the regulations and

(Ref 2) See "Further Education and the Nurse", N.B. Batley, Her Majesty's Inspector of Schools. Nursing Times 28 June 1968

"norms" of the institutions were respected. The methods adopted by a range of professions to ensure that courses in colleges, polytechnics and universities met their needs varied considerably, influenced to some extent by the degree of expertise available in the institutions themselves at different times. In the case of the Council, ultimate control was retained by a system of approval and re-approval which allowed for a large measure of flexibility within the prescribed requirements. Additionally, the Professional Advisers formed an essential link between the Council and the institutions; and this personal method of communication was supplemented by the provision of a "Hand-book" and other documents which were issued from time to time. The Council also made rules for the appointment by institutions of External Examiners and asked to be informed of their names. This particular arrangement was a modification of the method adopted in earlier days when the Council itself employed all External Examiners.

Theoretically, a general change in educational policy as a whole could also have jeopardised Health Visitor education; or, in individual cases, a major change in one institution could threaten a small development such as the Health Visitor course. In the one individual case where such a change was contemplated, care was taken by the Council to ensure that arrangements were made for the provision of student places elsewhere, in the tradition of the practice in institutions of Higher and Further Education. In general, educational policies had encouraged the developments of applied social science departments in recent years and the Council has taken advantage of this trend.

The debates on Devolution (see Section 4) were of considerable concern to the Council. The issues were referred in the first place to the Council's Advisory Committees for Wales and Scotland respectively for their comments and their reports were placed before Council in July 1978. The agreed statement by the Council that followed repeated the message that had come from all quarters, which was that Health Visitor Education and Training should continue to be organised on a U.K. basis.

It is self evident that a U.K. organisation could not have ignored any substantial changes which might have arisen out of the Devolution debates (Ref 3). In the event, however, no radical changes were made, and on the basis of the evidence from the National Advisory Committees to Council, it appeared that the efforts of the Council throughout its history in trying to preserve a balance between maintaining comparable standards in courses overall and, at the same time, making allowances for the differences that exist between the four countries, could claim to have been generally successful.

(Ref 3) "Our Changing Democracy - Devolution to Scotland and Wales 1975". HMSO Cmnd 6348
"Devolution the English Dimension". HMSO 1976

The links between the Council and the Health and Education Departments respectively were maintained by the system of Assessors. This method proved very satisfactory in so far as it allowed for a two way flow of information and for formal and informal consultation and advice. The appointment of the representatives of the Government Departments as assessors, rather than members who could vote had a double advantage. On the one hand it allowed the Council complete freedom to exercise its statutory powers; and on the other it avoided the embarrassment which might otherwise have been caused to such representatives in the event of any disagreement arising betweeen a Government Department and the Council.

The Influence of Related Professions

The extent to which the development of one profession is affected by the presence and the development of another could form the basis of a separate study. It will be readily agreed, however, that the work carried out by nurses in hospital varies very much in different parts of the world, partly because of the activities of other related professions, which suggests that this may be one of the main reasons for the difficulty of defining nursing on a world-wide basis. Recent negotiations within the European Economic Community had revealed substantial differences between the countries comprising the Community. While the Briggs Report had recommended "that Colleges of Nursing and Midwifery shall be established" and the preparations for the 1979 Act suggested close association between Nursing and Midwifery in legal terms, in France, for example, they were seen as quite separate professions. By the same token it might be suggested that no exact counterpart of the Health Visitor can be found in the other countries in the Community, although there are a number of workers carrying out similar functions in many places. Much variation is seen also in Health Visitor practice even within the United Kingdom where one individual may be engaged in a specialised aspect of Health Visiting only, such as Geriatric Care, another will undertake the full range of duties from 'cradle to grave' and another may combine Health Visiting duties with those of District Nursing and Midwifery, influenced by the presence (or otherwise) of other workers. The influence of other professions will also vary from time to time. The burgeoning of the Social Work profession in the 1960's and early 1970's was of immediate interest to the Council, not only because of the domestic problems of overcrowding that arose as a result of the increase in staff of the Central Council for the Education and Training in Social Work within the premises which it shared with the Council, but also because the expansion of Social Work itself

- for example in connection with child welfare policy - and the practical support afforded by the Government Departments to the development of Social Work appeared to threaten the very foundation of Health Visiting itself. During the Middle Years, however, the relative positions of both professions became more clearly understood and the Council's attention turned to the effect of the discontinuation of the profession of Medical Officer of Health, the changes in General Practice including the effect of the work of the Royal College of General Practitioners and, more recently, the efforts to enhance the education and training and the position of District Nurses.

This last development can also be used to illustrate the effect of one profession upon another. In 1980, the Panel of Assessors for District Nurse Training published a new Syllabus for District Nurse Education and Training after receiving, together with others, comments from the Council in 1977 which had included the suggestion that "While the expertise of District Nurses and Health Visitors is different, there are areas of common interest" and that "it would be reasonable to explore the possibility of a common core - the Council would be pleased to explore this subject further." As courses for the District Nurses and Health Visitors increasingly became established alongside each other in institutions of Higher and Further Education, a joint statement was issued in September 1980 by the two responsible bodies giving guidance for considerations to be borne in mind by those arranging these two types of course (Ref 4). In this case, the immediate stimulus for action arose on educational grounds as the possibility of shared learning became a practical issue in the institutions offering both courses. Therefore, in spite of the inbuilt difficulties arising from the fact that the two courses were of different duration, and that the new District Nurse syllabus as yet untried, it seemed necessary to clarify the educational issues involved as early as possible. To some extent history was repeating itself, since it had been difficult in earlier years to find ways of collaborating between the Health Visitor course of one year and the Social Work course of two years duration, especially while the Generic Social Work Course was still in the early stages of its development.

Recognition that professional attitudes may be formed for good or ill at the student stage had become more widespread and, while the form of joint studies amongst student groups concerned with Primary Care still remained at the experimental stage, and might receive low priority in what were often overcrowded timetables, the climate for encouraging mutual understanding had become more favourable, as those who have experienced interprofessional attitudes over two decades can testify.

(Ref 4) Panel of Assessors for District Nurse Training and Council for the Education and Training of Health Visitors - Discussion Paper "Health Visitor and District Nurse Courses - A Question of Shared Learning"

The symposium on interprofessional learning in Nottingham in 1979 (Ref 5), which was organised in equal partnership between the Royal College of General Practitioners, The Panel of Assessors, The Central Council for Education and Training in Social Work and the CETHV, demonstrated for the first time the official commitment of these bodies to the concept of thinking together. The symposium was the latest in a series of events, in which the Council had played a prominent role over the years, which were aimed at the promotion of better understanding between the professions engaged in Primary Health Care.

This symposium also exemplified the extent of the Council's interest in both areas of curative nursing and of primary care. This two-directional pull towards co-operation with nurses engaged in hospital care on the one hand and with those professionals engaged in primary health care on the other caused tension at times, but to have totally committed energies in one direction could only have been achieved at the expense of the other. To give opportunities to explain the Council's views and activities and to allow discussion, "Open Days" for Nurse Managers and later for Directors of Nursing Education were held in England and/or Scotland each summer.

Added to these was the extensive range of conferences based on the publication "An Investigation into the Principles of Health Visiting". (Ref 6). The comments of speakers and others on this document were subsequently incorporated in a further publication, "The Investigation Debate". (Ref 7).

Throughout its history the Council had encouraged Health Visitor students to undertake joint learning with other student groups and to make greater use of the wide range and variety of facilities available in institutions of Higher and Further Education. For clearly the Health Visitor students, as well as being aware of their colleagues in the hospital service and bearing in mind the knowledge and experience that they themselves had gained in this field, had now to give attention to a new working environment, a range of different professional colleagues and a different set of goals.

The Relationship between 'Education' and 'Service'

The establishment and maintenance of a satisfactory relationship between those responsible for the education of Health Visitors and those responsible for the service was a major consideration. Success in these relationships appeared to depend firstly on an appreciation of relative roles, secondly on the provision of constant and effective communications and thirdly on the discussion of matters of mutual

(Ref 5) "Education for co-operation in Health and Social Work", publ. The Journal of the Royal College of General Practitioners
(Ref 6) "An Investigation into the Principles of Health Visiting", pub. CETHV 1977
(Ref 7) "The Investigation Debate," pub. CETHV 1980

interest. No doubt too there must be a personal factor in this never-ending task. Without these provisions, those involved in education and training could soon become isolated from the realities of the service and those in the service would lose touch with the aims and objectives of the courses. If such situations were allowed to develop there would be a loss of confidence between the two parties ultimately leading to the ineffectiveness or even the discontinuation of individual courses. It is to the credit of all concerned, not least some of the Nurse Managers who were unfamiliar with Health Visiting and to the continuing efforts of Health Visitor Tutors, that the cases of loss of confidence that came to the attention of the Council were very rare indeed. It was evident too that the benefits of close association could be mutual. Tutors gained much from their frequent visits to and discussions with Service Managers, usually in more than one authority, while those in the Service gained from the stimulation of new ideas emanating from the courses. In the last analysis, of course, each is dependent upon the other.

As far as basic Health Visitor Courses are concerned, the responsibilities of the parties involved are broadly as follows :

The institutions of Higher and Further Education are responsible for the final selection of students and the arrangements for the courses. The Services are responsible for the sponsorship of students, the provision of Fieldwork Teachers, Assessors of Supervised Practice, and others who help in the practical training of students and for the ultimate employment of the qualified Health Visitor; and the Statutory Body is responsible for the approval of the courses. While the Council had agreed areas of responsibility, vis a vis the institutions of Higher and Further Education, further definition of responsibility for the interests of individual students had to be left to the local arrangements which were agreed between the institutions and the sponsoring authorities. Although this legal framework for the protection of all concerned was now more closely defined, equally important was the development of mutual understanding on a personal basis; and this was so effective that in practice the number of difficulties involving individual students that came to the notice of the Council were very few.

The Council attempted to initiate and encourage mutual understanding in a number of different ways. Firstly by visits by the Council's Professional Advisers to Institutions and Service Managers, and secondly by arranging "Open Days" for Managers, Fieldwork Teachers' conferences and by providing a range of publications. The recognition of the importance of the role of the service personnel in the preparation of the student Health Visitor was emphasised in the

Council's requirement for written evidence of the arrangements made for the provision of practical work facilities before a Health Visitor course was approved and, also, in the involvement of Service Managers and Fieldwork Teachers during the official "Visitations" to Institutions.

The increasing attention paid by the Council over the years to the preparation of the Fieldwork Teachers underlined its belief that they hold a key position in preparing the Health Visitor. Their understanding of the theoretical instruction in the course could help the student avoid the potential danger of dissociating theory and practice; and their attitudes, the state of their morale and the way they carried out their tasks could have a lasting effect on students who were often taking their first tentative steps away from the structured work within an institution to the less clearly defined and often disturbing role of community worker.

The membership of Council included representatives of Nurse Management and, in addition, others representing the Services were co-opted to serve on working parties on a number of occasions. In these and many other ways, contact was maintained between the Council and the Service but, nevertheless, there was always the danger that it would be thought, rightly or wrongly, that a Statutory Body concerned with education and training was out of touch with the needs and practices of the Service. Following some criticism arising from the Council's report on Fieldwork Teacher courses, more attention was given to the circulation of consultative documents before further new courses were established. The comments received, however, were revealing and displayed very wide differences of opinion among the Service Managers themselves at different levels. Similarly, there were differing views from different localities on the required content of the Health Visitor courses. These differences may be explained in some instances by ineffective communication and inadequate understanding. For example, there was some difficulty in finding a way of keeping in touch with the Regional Nursing Officers as a group. When eventually the Council's Director obtained an invitation to attend their meeting, it became evident that with some exceptions they were less well informed about and sympathetic to the Council's business as a whole than were the Chief Administrative Nursing Officers and Area Nursing Officers who were sponsoring health visitor students and with whom the Professional Advisers had frequent contact. Arrangements were subsequently made, therefore, for a representative of the Regional Nursing Officers to have discussions with the Council's Director twice a year and for a report of these meetings to be submitted to the meetings of the Regional Nursing Officers.

While some differences of views on Health Visiting could be accounted for by differences in levels of interest and understanding as well as by the extraordinary variations in conditions throughout the community, the Council's policy in relation to the Health Visitor course itself has remained consistent. The Health Visitor course must be both basic and general and, while account must be taken of the demands of the moment both locally and nationally, these must not be allowed unduly to distort the basic studies. If follows from this that employing authorities might need to give considerable attention to the induction of new members of staff and the provision of extra training where exceptional "Specialised" duties are required. While it is fully expected that those involved in the practices of the profession should have an influence upon training (a tradition dating back to Florence Nightingale's time when the matron was in charge of the nursing school and manifested again in modern times by the major influence of the Nurse Administrators on the formation of the 1979 Act) only comparatively recently has the question been raised of the contribution that those involved in education and training might make to the planning of the service. Yet it is possible to make out a strong case for such a contribution and, on a local basis, it already appears that an increasing number of Health Visitor tutors and other staff from institutions are being invited to serve as members of Health Authorities. This in turn could forge yet another link between the Institutions and the Service. The conclusions reached in the study undertaken by Alison McClymont (Ref 8) was that on the small sample taken, Health Visitors found on the whole that courses they had attended, while not necessarily geared to the specific needs of a particular district, had prepared them generally for the wide-ranging duties Health Visitors are called upon to perform. On occasion, however, there were complaints that this was not so, and it would be logical in any such case, therefore, to suggest a two-pronged investigation. Could the Health Visitor Course have been made more relevant or was it that the management failed to offer a suitable environment for the Health Visitors to carry out their tasks? Various debates between educational staff and service managers that have occurred in the course of the Council's work suggest these could lead to the profitable generation of ideas. While the ultimate responsibilities and skills of each party must be respected, there was reason to suppose that the challenge and counter challenge provided here and in the wider circle of higher and further education stimulated progress and ensured the avoidance of stagnation or dogmatism. This in turn, it is hoped, resulted in improvements in courses and, subsequently, in the provision of a better service.

(Ref 8) "Teaching for Reality", Alison McClymont, pub. CETHV 1980

Internal Changes—The appointment of the 4th Chairman and the 6th Council and the responsibilities of members

In 1977, Dr. Clifford Butler, Vice-Chancellor of the University of Loughborough, took over the Chairmanship of the Council from Professor (now Sir John) Butterfield. The Council has been particularly fortunate in having two such eminent men as Chairmen at times when width of experience and objectivity of views were of particular value. The fifth Council concluded its terms of office in June 1977, the sixth Council with two-thirds new members was appointed to serve from October 1977 onwards. Before the three year term was due to be concluded, the members were invited to continue in office until such time as the Council should cease to exist. With three exceptions, all members accepted this invitation.

In an age when it is widely accepted that members of Councils and Committees should be elected by the democratic process, the appointment of members on the lines of the schedule of the 1962 Act which allowed only for nominations may seem to be an anachronism. Be that as it may, to those who work for the Council it has been clear that the breadth of knowledge and expertise of these nominated members has been invaluable to the Council which itself has provided the opportunity for the results of the meeting of very different minds to be brought to bear on the business of the Education and Training of Health Visitors. Understandably, the Health Visitor tutors, who along with others holding Health Visitor qualifications comprised about a third of the membership, had to take a major part in most aspects of the work of a Council responsible for education and training and individual Health Visitor tutors especially were known to have made as many as 25 to 30 attendances a year on Council business. This suggests that a slight change in the ratio of Health Visitor members to non-Health Visitors might have spread the load. At the same time, however, many other members who were not Health Visitors gave very generously of their time. The overall total of meetings reached 80 in 1979 when rapid developments were taking place and, apart from some suggestion for comparatively slight adjustment of work between committee and working party and/or more cross-membership between Committees, (for example, "Qualifications" and "Professional Development") at no time were there complaints to the author that a meeting had been ineffective or unnecessary. While it was only to be expected that Health Visitor members themselves would give full support to their own Council, sometimes even at considerable cost to themselves, the attendance of the other members was equally impressive. These other members did not merely attend meetings in a passive role, but brought their diverse knowledge and skills to bear as fully active and involved participants. The resulting mixture of experience and viewpoints provided a wholly beneficial, if sometimes uncomfortable, element of challenge and questioning into the work of the Council.

The Structure of the Council's Staff

The Middle Years saw a number of changes in the composition and membership of the Council's staff. The first Chief Professional Adviser, later Director, Elaine Wilkie, retired in April 1975 and her place was taken by the author. When the separation from the CCETSW took place in 1974, all the senior members of the Joint Administrative Staff moved over to the larger Social Work Council and the Health Visitor Council was faced with the task of appointing new staff according to the "establishment" prescribed by the DHSS and, with the appointment of the first Principal Administrative Officer in the Spring of 1975, new administrative procedures had to be devised. Throughout the Middle Years, the post of Principal Professional Adviser was created within the "cash limits" by reducing persistent problem arising from the different salary scales in operation for various grades of staff. This difficulty added particularly to the load of the Director, the Principal Administrative Officer and the Professional Advisers themselves. The ratio of professional to administrative staff, approximately one to two, proved slightly out of balance and, with the approval of the DHSS, one further post of Professional Adviser was created within the "cash limits" by reducing the number of junior administrative staff. The final total therefore became nine professional staff including the Director and twenty administrative staff.

The demands of the Council's on-going and developmental work, the preparation of comments, the liaison with the service and institutions and other activities were found to be placing an increasing load on the staff, and following a detailed study of assignments and work loads, the "case" for an increase of up to fifteen Professional Advisers and the appropriate equivalent increase in administration staff was accepted by the Finance and General Purpose Committee in June 1977. By this time however, the work of the "Co-ordinating Committee" was under way. As this Committee, at the direction of the Minister of State (Health), was charged with the task of preparing for new legislation which would replace the provisions of the 1962 Act, the matter was taken no further. Nevertheless, it is noteworthy that the work of the Council's staff had become so extensive that, in the opinion of the Council, a substantial increase in staff would have been justified.

The Relationship between Council Members and Council Staff

Much has been written about the relationship between MPs and Civil Servants. In microcosmic form, the relationship between Council members and Council staff had some of the same features. Firstly, power must lie ultimately in the hands of the Council members and it was the business of the Council staff to ensure that members received the necessary information on which to base their decisions and then to see that the policies and actions required by the Council were carried out. Here, however, those who held the power, i.e. the members, could only devote a fraction of their time to the work of the Council. Furthermore with as short a time as three years in office, in some cases extended to a second and more rarely to a third term, they were necessarily dependent upon the staff not only for information but frequently for guidance. It was the staff, therefore, who to a substantial degree, provided continuity in the business of the Council. This was always apparent when a new Council was appointed and particularly so in 1977. In that year two-thirds of the members were new-comers and in an extreme case a Committee might have to be reappointed with little if any continuity of membership. The briefing by the staff, which was routinely made available to Chairmen before meetings, had in these cases to be considerably elaborated, incidentally adding to the responsibilities of the staff concerned. Thus the arrangements for the appointment of Council as prescribed in the 1962 Act which did not make provisions for phased changes of membership was shown to have this deficiency which could also have been a source of embarrassment - for example, if the members of the sixth Council, which came into office at the height of the debate on the Nurses, Midwives and Health Visitors Bill, had taken a very different stance from that of their predecessors. In the event this did not occur. Moreover, while it is expected that a change of Government will mean a change of policy, there was an expectation that a statutory body such as the CETHV would demonstrate consistency.

The ways in which members and staff work together was of obvious importance and while the staff were employed and entrusted to carry out the day to day work of the Council, they had to ensure that the ultimate responsibility for all major decisions was left in the hands of the Council itself and those Committees to which it had delegated powers. Not infrequently, however, after an issue had been discussed by members, the further stages were left to the discretion of staff. For example, Council wished for some clarification on the ways in which 'comments from Council' were to be taken and it was left to the Director to devise a formula for Council to approve if they so wished.

Following the approval, it was left in her hands to use discretion on interpretation within the agreed formula.

However formalised the pattern of procedure might be, in the last analysis a great deal must depend upon relationships and on trust between Chairman and Council members and Council staff. Members could, and did, challenge the action taken by the staff or the content of papers prepared and, at the same time, staff saw it as their duty to point out possible consequences of suggestions made by members. While overall legal responsibilities under the Act remained the same, each Council developed its own style and the way it implemented the Act was shaped according to the abilities and interests of Council members and Council staff and their interaction.

The Work of the Council's Staff

The commonly heard arguments for and against the principal officer of an organisation being either a 'lay' administrator or a 'professional' again find some echoes in the history of the Council. Initially, the senior staff consisted of a triad, a Joint Secretary who worked for both the Social Work and the Health Visitor Councils and below him the two chief Professional Advisers heading up the two groups of professional staff. With the total separation of the two Councils in 1974 the Health Visitor Council decided "on a structure which would have a Director who was a Health Visitor supported by two Principal Officers, one concerned with administration and one with professional matters." Experience in the 'Middle Years' suggested, at least to the author, that the advantages of the new system were three-fold. Firstly as a Health Visitor the Director had an understanding of the practice and the education and training of the profession. Secondly the Director could readily appreciate the significance of changes in external circumstances which might affect the work of the Council and thirdly he/she should have the background knowledge on which to base decisions on priorities. Added to this, acceptance by the profession should be easier for someone who is known to have had experience in these fields and therefore could have some understanding of the situations and the problems faced by those employed in education and the service alike. The Director, however, in turn must rely upon the advice of the Principal Administrative Officer and the Principal Professional Adviser and undoubtedly the work of the Council was most effective when these top posts were filled and it was possible to consult together regularly at what became known as "triangle meetings".

The work of each Professional Adviser had three aspects. Firstly she was responsible for liaison within a defined geographical section of the U.K. visiting both the Educational Institutions and the Service Managers. To keep in touch with Regional Nursing Officers and CANO's and ANO's as well as to meet as many District Nursing Officers as possible was no small task. While in some cases it was evident that little was known about the community services and it was an uphill task to try to encourage Managers to be concerned with this area of work, the frequent response of "come again" could be taken as an indication of interests by others. At the same time, the Council gained inestimable advantages from the constant inflow of information from the field that was available in this way. Secondly, each Professional Adviser was assigned to one or more of the Council's committees and working parties; and thirdly each Adviser acted as a "resource person" on a particular subject or subjects. The policy of basing professional staff in the London office was continued with one exception as, in spite of the disadvantages of having to travel to different parts of the U.K., this pattern gave greater opportunities for the interchange of information and ideas between staff and allowed the desirable flexibility in relation to staff assignments without incurring either the problem of requiring staff to move house at intervals or the potential danger of leaving the geographical assignments of members of staff unchanged for year after year. The exception to the policy of centralisation was made in 1979 when a small office was eastablished in Edinburgh to act as a base for one member of the professional staff who was provided with part-time secretarial assistance. This small office also proved useful as a meeting place for teaching staff and service managers and helped in the development of the already well-established practice of liaison between the CETHV and the GNC (Scotland), the CMB (Scotland) and the Committee for Clinical Nursing Studies. With a total of six centres for Health Visitor Education and Training together with the problems of travel in the winter months, duties in Scotland were already taking up the equivalent of the time of one full-time member of the professional staff and this alone seemed to justify an exception to the rule of basing staff in London. The Council was given help both by the DHSS from whom the Council's funding was ultimately drawn, and from the SHHD in this new move. The full implications of this development have yet to be seen but undoubtedly it has proved to have had some of the advantages that were anticipated. But, in spite of every effort to keep in touch, the Professional Adviser concerned could not have the same everyday knowledge of developments at Headquarters as the other Advisers had; and there was also the inherent danger of some degree of national isolation occurring. In an attempt to prevent this occurring, the Professional Adviser concerned not only retained a small geographical assignment in England but she also attended Council and some Committee meetings and staff meetings, and had responsibility for some Committee work in London. Additionally, she was joined in Scotland by other Professional Advisers on those occasions when their knowledge as "resource" members of staff was required, and, of course, by senior members of staff for the meetings of the Scottish Advisory Committee and other groups.

The skills and the knowledge of the Professional Advisers must necessarily be at the heart of the work of a Council designed to deal with the education and training of Health Visitors and indeed, nearly every activity, other than those concerning administration only, involved the contribution of one or more members of the professional staff to a greater or lesser degree.

Together they contributed to the body of knowledge central to the on-going and developmental aspects of the Council's work without which the progress of Health Visitor education, as demonstrated throughout the history of the Council, could not have been sustained.

This emphasis on the key role of the professional staff in no way diminishes the importance of the role of the administrative staff since the work of both is naturally complementary. It took some time to accommodate to the new situation that arose when the Council gained full independence in 1974, but with the more experienced staff which it was now possible to attract to the administrative posts (reflecting the state of the labour market), it was possible to develop a much higher standard of minuting, record-keeping and general financial and office management, under the guidance of the Principal Administrative Officer, than had been possible hitherto. Usually it was obvious where the skills of professional staff and the skills of the administrative staff could best be used but, in a period of change, adjustments had to be made. Generally the trend was to relieve the professional staff of extraneous duties which they had undertaken in the past when only inadequate administrative support was available. Additionally, defined units, covering the Committee Secretariat, Records, Financial and Administrative work respectively, which it had been impracticable to establish in earlier years were organised. Throughout the Middle Years, Council had been fortunate in being served by staff who had been prepared to turn their hands to a variety of tasks as and when the need arose.

The Joint Staff Consultative Committee

With the 'establishment' of posts now filled, it became necessary early in 1975 to reconsider the 'Conditions of Service'. A joint Staff

Consultative Committee was therefore formally established by Council. Within its terms of reference was the right to report direct to the Council, but in practical terms it was found useful to associate the meetings of the JSCC with those of the Finance and General Purposes Committee. After considerable debate, new 'Conditions of Service' were prepared which were later passed by Council and forwarded for the approval of the DHSS. In addition to the formal JSCC meetings, a quarterly meeting of all staff, chaired by the Director, was arranged, to give an opportunity for progress reports on matters of general interest to be made and to allow discussion on matters raised by the staff themselves if they so wished. These arrangements appeared particularly necessary and were especially useful during a period of uncertainty when legal changes affecting the position of the Council and therefore of the Council's staff were pending.

The serious problems caused by the employment of staff on four different salary scales persisted throughout this 5 year period and with the full agreement and co-operation of staff the matter was referred for investigation by the appropriate section of the DHSS in an effort to rationalise the situation. The Finance and General Purposes Committee and the Joint Staff Consultative Committee were jointly of the opinion, however, that the Report produced did not offer the prospect of satisfactorily resolving the matter and the Department of Health was informed that "Council found itself unable to accept the conclusions reached."

Accommodation

The problems of accommodation at Clifton House were made acute by the rapid expansion of the CCETSW in the early 1970's and were exacerbated further by structural alterations to the fabric of the building initiated by the landlords in 1975 -1976. These problems were finally resolved when the Council moved into a new suite of modern offices on the fourth floor of Clifton House at the beginning of 1977. This development not only provided the Council for the first time with good working conditions, but also allowed it to present an appropriate 'image' to the many visitors from the U.K. and from overseas who made their way to the Council's offices. Before the final decision to stay at Clifton House was reached, a number of other office buildings were considered and one proposal, which would have allowed for the accommodation of the Council and one other of the existing bodies concerned with nursing education was put to the DHSS but was turned down on financial grounds. In the event, however, the excellence of the new offices within Clifton House coupled with the advantages of accessibility proved most satisfactory and the patient endurance of months of noise and dust worthwhile. Although some of the related statutory bodies have had the advantage of being housed in the dignity of 'listed' Buildings, from 1977 onwards the Council had the alternative practical advantage of being accommodated in a modern office block and to those who had experienced the discomforts of previous years in particular, this move provided a boost to morale, the means of improving efficiency and gave the Council a new standing and new opportunities for development.

SECTION 1 SUPPLEMENT 1

RECENT EVIDENCE OF THE DEMAND FOR THE HEALTH VISITING SERVICE

GOVERNMENT DEPARTMENT REPORTS

First report of The Social Services and Employment Sub-committee of The House of Commons Expenditure Committee.

"In 1974, the UK average ratio of health visitors to population was 1:5,822... We view this figure with concern, *and recommend that strenuous efforts should be made to improve on it.*"

Prevention and health: everybody's business. Health Departments of Great Britain and Northern Ireland.

"Most plans to prevent disease depend on health education of the public".

"Health education as practised by midwives, health visitors and school nurses has in the past been enormously successful ...."
"New initiatives .... are now needed ...."

Priorities for Health and Personal Social Services in England. Department of Health and Social Security

"............ the growth envisaged for the primary care services as a whole, and for health visitors in particular ...."

The Health Service in Scotland. The Way Ahead.
Scottish Home and Health Department

"the........ a continuation on a modest scale of the recent expansion in the number of health visitors".

Proposed All-Wales Policies for the Planning and Provision of Health & Social Services from 1976/77 to 1979/80. Welsh Office.

"The domiciliary services — particularly home nursing and health visiting — are extremely important to general preventive health and to the policy of maintaining vulnerable groups in the community......"

Strategy for the Development of Health and Personal Social Services in Northern Ireland.
Department of Health and Social Services

"The requirement............ is not simply for more district nurses, health visitors and other professional or ancillary workers. It is to deploy total resources, present and future, to the best advantage''.

RECENT REPORTS

Court Report. Fit for the Future

Recommendation:— ''Within the community nursing services there should be a distinct group of nurses, called health visitors ....''

Snowdon Report. Integrating the Disabled

Recommendation:— ''That the health visitor should be the person who acts as the referral point for the disabled person..........''

Advisory Committee on Services for Hearing-Impaired People

''......we consider that the Health Visitor is the most suitable person to screen pre-school children..........''

First Report from the Select Committee on Violence in the Family. Session 1976-77. Violence to Children. para. 133

'' ....We are not in a position to say how the health visitor service best be organised. In reviewing the recommendations of the Court Report, DHSS should consider how health visitors can be most effectively deployed in any particular geographical area. What is important, however, is that there should be an adequate number of health visitors to cover all the needs of the community whether old or young. The Minister of State reminded us that the DHSS's consultative document ''Priorities for the Health and Social Services'' had envisaged a 6 per cent increase per annum in the number of health visitors. Cuts in Government expenditure made it uncertain whether that target would be achieved. **We recommend that this target should be achieved''.**

SECTION 2

THE EXERCISE OF POWERS

The Council continued to exercise the statutory functions ascribed to it under the 1962 provisions which had proved to have considerable advantages but some limitations.

The uses made of these powers during the Middle Years are described in general terms under three headings, followed by a record of the results of the Strategy Exercise of 1975.

The Legal Framework

The functions of the Council are laid down in the 1962 Act in the following terms:

"(a) shall promote the training of health visitors by seeking to secure suitable facilities for the training of persons intending to become health visitors, by approving courses as suitable to be attended by such persons and by seeking to attract persons to such courses;

(b) if it appears to them that adequate provision is not being made for the further training of health visitors, shall provide or secure the provisions of courses for this purpose;

(c) may conduct or make arrangements for the conduct of examinations in connection with such courses as are mentioned in the preceding paragraphs; and

(d) may carry out or assist other persons in carrying out research into matters relevant to the training of health visitors."

It is self evident that the work of any statutory body is controlled by the wording of the relevant Act or Acts relating to its establishment and by any further definitions contained in any subsequent "Rules" and "Statutory Instruments". In this instance, two additional Statutory Instruments were added, namely:

1971 No. 1221 (C.31)
LOCAL AUTHORITY SOCIAL SERVICES
The Local Authority Social Services Act 1970
(Commencement No. 3) Order 1971

1971 No. 1241
SOCIAL SERVICES
The Central Council for Education and Training in Social
Work Order 1971

The clear and definitive wording of the 1962 Act continued to provide the Council with the opportunity to develop all aspects of Health Visitor education and training throughout the U.K., and apart from the mounting concern felt over the omission of disciplinary powers, there is no evidence to suggest that the Council of its own volition would have wished to instigate radical change in its responsibilities. In practical terms, the 1962 Act provided an exceptionally wide range of 'functions' spanning recruitment, the stipulation of prerequisite qualifications for admission to courses, the provision and approval of Health Visitor courses, and the development of further education and research. From the experience of the Council, it was clear that it was this exceptional range of responsibilities together with related developments, that generated the volume of work, which was characteristic of the "Middle Years".

The omission of a disciplinary function from the 1962 Act meant that the Council was empowered to award a certificate, which in effect became a licence to practise, but that it had no powers to take away a certificate once awarded or to maintain a register from which names could be removed. Stimulated partly by the case of a Health Visitor's misdemeanour which was brought to the attention of the Council, a Working Party was set up to investigate the matter in June 1977. As an interim measure, the Principal Administrative Officer wrote to all employing authorities to ensure they were aware of the situation described above and asking for any information about "cases" which appeared to require disciplinary procedures which came to their attention. The anonymous information provided in response to this request together with a study of procedures adopted by other professional bodies, enabled a draft 'Memorandum and Code of Practice' to be submitted to Council in January 1979; and this was sent to the relevant professional organisations for comment in the first instance. As the subject of disciplinary procedures was outside the terms of the 1962 Act, particular care was taken to ensure that this work was instigated only with the full knowledge and agreement of the Government Departments' Assessors. This matter subsequently became more urgent in view of the progress which was being made towards the passing of the 1979 Act which, it was understood, would include provision for disciplinary procedures for Health Visitors as well as for Nurses and Midwives. A second, but easily remedied omission from the 1962 Act concerned the provisions for National Advisory Committees. The Act had established Advisory Committees for Scotland and Northern Ireland (in slightly different terms), but had omitted any similar mention of Wales and England. It is presumed this was in keeping with the political situation of that time. The Council, however, was able to make good these omissions by the simple device of establishing as committees of Council itself first in 1975 a National Advisory Committee for Wales and later in 1980 a National Advisory Committee for England. Both of these Committees were serviced not by the Health Departments of the Countries concerned but by the Council's staff.

In 1975, the Council was beginning to express an interest in planning courses for school nurses and this provided an opportunity for testing the interpretation of the Act. The involvement of Health Visitors in the school nursing service had a very long history, a substantial proportion of Health Visitors in the past having had work in schools included in their duties. Indeed, as far back as 1954, it had been officially suggested that eventually all school nurses should hold the Health Visitor's Certificate. While this suggestion was never implemented, many Health Visitors were actively concerned with the health of the schoolchild and there were substantial reasons therefore for the Council's involvement in the education and training of school nurses. Before this development could take place, however, the legal basis for such a move had to be referred in the first instance to the DHSS, as this Department already dealt with the joint financing of, and other joint administrative matters concerning, the Council; and direct correspondence with other Health Departments became necessary at a later stage because the establishment of courses in School Nursing had to take account of the variations in national policies. The Situation that eventually emerged is described in Section 4.

In general, however, the history of the Council reflected the implementation of a well-constructed and well-worded Act. A document such as the Act, which is legally binding, is naturally of fundamental importance. At the same time, it must be remembered that its interpretation and implementation rested in the hands of Council members and Council staff. And while history cannot show how the functions would have been discharged had they been implemented by different individuals, the record as it stands show that a substantial volume of activity had by now been taken in respect of each of the Council's functions; and that this included much which had been remarked on by other bodies as being of an innovatory and pioneering nature.

The Work of the Council, the Committees and Working Parties

(See Section 2 Supplement 1)

The methods by which the Council undertook its work continued in accordance with the plan described in "The History of the Council for the Education and Training of Health Visitors'' by Elaine Wilkie. Council meetings were normally held four times a year but additionally ''Extraordinary'' meetings were called during this period on the specific subjects of Obstetric Courses, the Court Report, and the Nurses, Midwives and Health Visitors Bill respectively. The pattern of holding one meeting every second year outside London in Scotland, Wales or Northern Ireland was also continued. These meetings, however, were considerably more expensive than those held in London and for this reason on one occasion this practice was not followed. At the meetings away from the London Headquarters, members of the appropriate National Advisory Committee were invited to attend as observers in order further to encourage understanding throughout the U.K. of an organisation which was in practical terms largely London based.

The agenda of Council meetings generally started with major policy matters followed by the reports of the National Advisory Committees (see Section 4) and of the five main committees of Council: ''Education'', ''Qualifications'', ''Professional Development'' (i.e. further education), ''Research'' and ''Finance and General Purposes''. The business was then debated and specific decisions were made by Council, where required, on the basis of the written reports included with Council papers and the oral reports made by the Chairpersons. Each committee worked to ''terms of reference'' approved by the Council which directed their activities and delegated powers to them; the terms of reference themselves were modified by Council from time to time as was found necessary. Each committee could and frequently did form working groups to undertake particular pieces of work, such as the design of courses for Assessors of Supervised Practice (Professional Development Committee) and a study of prerequisite qualifications for those entering Health Visitor courses (Education Committee). The Curriculum Development Working Party, first organised as a working group of Education Committee, was later reconstituted to include representatives from all the main committees of Council as the complex and comprehensive nature of its work became apparent. In 1976, Professor Butterfield decided to form a group of the Chairman of all the main committees to meet for an hour before each Council meeting with the following terms of reference: ''to formulate and submit to Council a cohesive policy regarding both external and internal developments in Council's work both for the short and long term.'' The ''Chairman's Committee,'' later expanded by Dr. Butler to include the chairman of the National Advisory Committees, proved to be a controversial development and Council members continued to express concern lest this group became ipso facto, a decision making body usurping the responsibilities of Council itself. The Chairman of Council, therefore, was required to report to the Council on all the matters discussed at its meetings, which included such topics as the consideration of the establishment of an office in Scotland, the fall in recruitment and priorities for the future. While there were potentially clear advantages in the existence of a forum of this nature, not least to the Director who could bring to the attention of the Chairpersons the magnitude of the demands made "in toto" upon the staff, this innovation, superimposed upon the original structure of the main committees, continued to present difficulties, notably in the attainment of a clearly defined and acceptable role. With Council members coming from all quarters of the UK with occupations as diverse as those of H.V.T. , Local Councillor and Polytechnic Director it was not unusual for a discussion at Council meetings to erupt suddenly into a lively exchange of views, and the subject of the Chairman's Committee, for example, provided a never-failing spur to controversy.

Apart from administrative matters concerning finance, staffing and accommodation, which were dealt with by Finance and General Purposes Committee, the business of the other main committees arose naturally out of the functions listed in the 1962 Act. The Education Committee dealt with the approval of a basic Health Visitor course including examination arrangements; Qualifications Committee was involved in individual matters concerning entry to Health Visitor, Fieldwork Teacher and Health Visitor Tutor courses and applications from abroad; Professional Development Committee was concerned with further education and Research Committee with in-house data collection and the stimulation and co-ordination of research concerning Health Visitor education and training. Council members were given the opportunity to indicate on which committees they would wish to serve; and while some adjustments had to be made to ensure proper representation on each committee, on average each Council member served on two committees and often on the related working parties. The number of co-opted members of each committee was determined by Council and in each case did not exceed one-third of the total membership. In these circumstances, Council was empowered to delegate various of its functions to the different committees in such a way that Council members remained in control of all the Council's business. This arrangement was conducive to consistency of policy throughout the lifetime of any one Council. The question of consistency of policy continuing from one Council to the next arose in particular at the meetings of Qualifications Committee where there had been a complete change of Chairman and membership when the new Council came into office in 1977.

On the one hand CETHV needed to show some consistency in policy over the years, for example over entry requirements to a course, while on the other hand members of the new Council would naturally wish to bring forward new ideas. In these cases the Professional Adviser of the committee, and, when appropriate, the Director and/or the Principal Officers had a responsibility to inform the committee of past history and to point out the implications of any radical changes in policy.

The number of Working Groups any one committee could 'carry' had to be limited for practical reasons. Exceptionally, Professional Development Committee at one time had no fewer than three working groups studying the subjects of Further Education, courses in School Nursing and courses for the Assessors of supervised Practice. It was here particularly that the services of co-opted members were required, not only to widen the collective knowledge of the group but also to spread the load of work which had become unduly heavy for some Council members. In practice, the plans and recommendations of working groups were by and large accepted by the parent committees and incorporated in reports forwarded for the attention of Council. Here again, the majority of reports on special subjects were approved by Council, although suggestions for modifications were not uncommon and referral back to the committee for further consideration not unknown.

Some of the Council's responsibilities did not fall so clearly into the remit of any of the main committees. "Attracting persons into such courses," in other words recruitment, had a chequered history and passed from the responsibility of the first "Development and Recruitment Committee" in the early years, later to the Chairman's Committee for oversight and eventually was added to the terms of reference of Education Committee. The subject of recruitment had continued to be a special responsibility of one Professional Adviser; it was constantly raised by all the Professional Advisers on their visits throughout the United Kingdom, and the recruitment position reported annually to Council in the form of a "Student Intake Analysis". With the benefit of hindsight, the failure to ensure that the same measure of attention was given to this subject as to other topics by a designated committee of Council may be attributed to the failure of the author, coming as she did from a different sphere of work, to appreciate the full effect on Health Visitor recruitment of the Reorganisation of the National Health Service in 1974. It seemed clear, however, that only by allocating the various functions defined in the Act as the particular responsibilities of the different Committees of Council could it be ensured that they received full and continuing attention.

Certain other activities were adapted or were established in the light of changing circumstances. The original sub-committee on "Medical and Nursing Management" was disbanded and eventually was recast with a different membership. This new formation, the Professional Organisations Consultative Committee, which consisted of repesentatives of related professional organisations based in England and in Scotland, evolved into a useful forum for the exchange of information and views on matters of mutual interest. Indeed, this newly formed and apparently unique group developed to the extent of producing in the spring of 1980, at the instigation of a member, a Resolution giving the consensus of the signatories on the subject of the new plans for the National Health Service. This somewhat unconventional action had to be clearly labelled "signed in a personal capacity" to ensure that no one had committed the organisation they represented. Indeed, as the group expanded to give wider representation it gained a momentum of its own. The Council's plan for Manpower Studies was criticised and challenged and further explanation demanded, and the representative of the Association of Nurse Managers had views to express on the financial problems faced by her colleagues in meeting the growing demand for further education. The Committee members themselves took the business of the meeting beyond the original terms of reference for it appeared that the Council had provided a new meeting place where those involved in events concerning the HV profession from 'north and south of the border' could deliberate frankly in a relaxed atmosphere. At these meetings it was found that the various actions by the individual bodies did not always meet with universal approval; nevertheless these occasions allowed the opportunity for explanations of action which could prevent misunderstandings caused solely by ignorance of the facts.

Other less formal activities instigated by the staff in the first instance, but supported generously by Council members on certain occasions, included "Open days" for Service Managers and later for Directors of Nursing Education each summer, and the author's meetings with groups of Health Visitor Tutors in five centres in the United Kingdom twice a year. These meetings were conducted informally, the Tutors themselves raising any subject they wished for discussion. The underlying purpose of all these meetings was to improve communications in both directions and to allow for mutual learning, for in the last analysis the Council depended on the skills and on the goodwill of those engaged in the service and of the teaching staff and it was the quality of their work which would decide the success or failure of the conversion of Council's policies into practice.

Ongoing Commitments, Areas of Development and Matters Arising out of External Changes.

The work of the Council overall can be considered in three inter-related categories: ongoing commitments, areas of development and matters arising out of external changes. Into the first category, for example, falls the business of the approval and reapproval of courses which, once started, provides an ongoing obligation, not least because of the involvement of the resources of both the Education and the Health Services. Areas of development can be defined as changes in established procedure as well as innovatory measures which add a new dimension to the Council's work. Each of the innovatory developments followed the three stages of a) planning, b) establishment and c) assessment and modification if required, a process which might span, very approximately, a five-year period. The third category, matters arising out of external changes, could hardly have been more fundamental, including as it did the effects of the 1974 Reorganisation, the EEC Directives concerning Nurse and Midwifery Training and the birth of the 1979 Act.

The Strategy Plan and Sequels

The final separation from the Social Work Council at the end of 1974, and the introduction of a number of new members of staff in the spring of 1975, provided a suitable moment for a review of work accomplished so far, and of a consideration of work still to be done. The first paper, "The Strategy Plan," on this subject was produced as the result of meetings of the senior staff in the first instance for the benefit of the staff themselves and, while exceptional pressure of business prevented the establishment of a systematic pattern of reviews, the theme was taken up in various papers to the Chairman's Committee and to the Council at intervals. This plan to meet a timetable of short-term and long-term action was found to have had considerable effect when it was reported to Council in the summer of 1980 that all the principal items listed in 1975 had received attention (see Section 2 Supplement 2).

The story of the Council's activities was one of continuing change and development for "as one door has opened another seven have been revealed." Clearly the pace and amount of work this generated at any one time was important and, while there was no evidence of stagnation in any department, it is known that undue pressure was felt on occasions by Council members and staff and by Health Visitor

Tutors. The uncertainties of the future legislation alone had provided extra impetus for the Council to accelerate plans while able still to use the existing statutory powers.

Comments from Council

The "Middle Years" produced a large number of reports which had relevance to the interests of the Council and providing "comments" proved to be a very substantial and time consuming commitment. In 1975, it appeared to be necessary for the Council to consider the overall policy to be adopted and a formula was devised for dealing with these reports of varying importance to the Council, ranging from a letter from the Director to the involvement of working parties of Council representatives, first nationally, then centrally, and "comments from Council" now became a standing item on the Council's Agenda. On occasions issues of prime importance were given a half session at the regular Council meeting for debate, and more rarely an extraordinary meeting of Council was called.

The ultimate effect of these comments cannot be estimated, but it appeared that in some cases even the strongly expressed views on very pertinent issues relating to the future of Council business were passed over, for example Council's views on the proposals for the 1979 Act, whilst in others they have been seen to have made an impression. The Council was particularly pleased to note the very favourable mention it received in the "Hospital and Social Service Journal" of the constructive comments it had made on the document concerning the suggested changes in the National Health Service (Ref 10). These suggestions included ideas on changing the focus of health care from Hospital to Community. The scope of the subjects covered in these reports, and the essence of the Council's comments, were indicative of the interests and of the policies of the Council. This suggested that the comparative study of these alongside the comments of other nursing and midwifery bodies, as well as those of other professions, would reveal significant ways in which professions think alike or where they differ. The Council has welcomed these opportunities to offer comments although the volume of work entailed was considerable for members and for staff alike. As a U.K. body, the Council was concerned in some cases with five separate but co-ordinated exercises - for example in connection with the proposed changes in the National Health Service four national and one central - and in other cases individual comments on the concerns of one country alone required attention (Ref 11). Where appropriate, the National Advisory

(Ref 10) 'Patients First' DHSS
'The Structure and Management of the National Health Service in Scotland'
'The Structure and Management of the Health and Personal Social Services in Northern Ireland'

(Ref 11) "Adoption of Children in Northern Ireland"

Committees prepared the first paper and, following Council's approval, comments were forwarded in the name of the Council. Where U.K. matters as a whole were concerned Working Groups with representatives from all four countries prepared the paper whenever possible, although for purely practical reasons it was not always so easy to get representation from Northern Ireland and Wales as it was from England and Scotland where there were a larger number of members to call upon. All Council members, however, had the opportunity to speak at Council meetings to the draft comments on all major issues before they were agreed. The policy of the Council, which emerged from the text of the comments, showed a commitment to the importance of a preventive service; to Health Visitor education and training and associated courses for Health Visitors and for School Nurses developing within a system of Higher and Further Education; to the desirability of associating with other staff and students of professions engaged in primary care and in unrelated spheres of work and to the aim that the basic course should prepare the Health Visitor for general duties in the first instances for adaptation to different localities and at different points in time. There was also a strong commitment to continuing education throughout professional life.

The Council's policy concerning the specialist Health Visitor was not quite so definite although the provision of specialist courses was taken up in the reports on further education. This issue may continue to be raised as the particular value of Health Visitors who have taken an extra course in, for example, diabetes or disabilities, has been mentioned in a number of quarters. And, of course, liaison between the Hospital services and the former Local Health Authorities by specialist HVs has a long history. The Council's hesitation may have been due to the very real problem that a diversion of Health Visitors to specialist activities could only be at the expense of an already undermanned general service and, also, that the less tangible aspects concerning prevention could easily be submerged in the obvious demands of after-care services. As the administration pattern emerging from the Reorganisation of the NHS in 1974 had placed the Health Visitor in closer proximity to the curative services - the danger of the preventive role being submerged had in any case become more serious.

Although the Council was frequently asked to comment on service matters this had to be avoided as it was outside the scope of the provisions of the 1962 Act. Correspondents were advised, therefore, to write to either their Professional Organisation or the appropriate Health Department.

The Extending Responsibilities.

While those concerned with the first phase of the Council's history had managed with very limited resources to design a new pattern of Health Visitor education and established new policies and new standards, those involved in the "Middle Years" had two dominant preoccupations. First of all they carried on the functions as required under the 1962, Act, building on the foundations already laid, at times adding a new dimension or taking a new initiative. Secondly, much attention had to be given perforce to the preparations for the 1979 Act. In the latter case, the Council continued throughout to pursue the two-fold policy of offering to co-operate with the Nurses and Midwives and at the same time requiring that the education and training of Health Visitors which had, by now, become successfully established in institutions of Higher and Further Education should be safeguarded.

Issues in health visitor training

Council for the Education and Training of Health Visitors

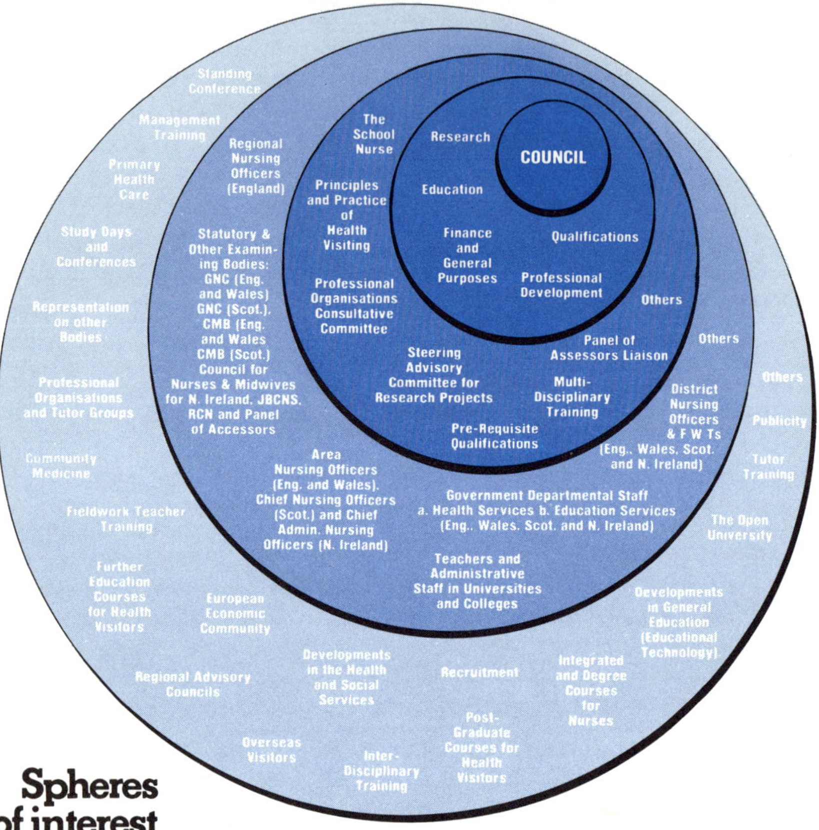

Spheres of interest

The Council

The Council, which was established under the Health Visiting and Social Work (Training) Act, 1962, is composed of a chairman appointed by the Privy Council and 31 members drawn from health visiting, nurse education, medicine, the health service and general education.

The Main Committees

The main committees are responsible to the Council regarding the statutory functions to 'promote the training of health visitors', 'approving courses', 'attracting persons to such courses', and the provision of 'further training for health visitors', 'make arrangements for the conduct of examinations', and 'carrying out or assisting other persons in the carrying out of research into matters relevant to the training of health visitors'.

Other Committees and Working Groups

Other committees and working groups are called to consider specific topics as they arise and to ensure communication with organisations with related interests.

Service Contacts (Health and Education)

The Council and the Council's staff are in contact continually with government departments, nursing organisations, with those responsible for the service throughout the United Kingdom and with the staffs of universities and colleges concerned with courses.

Other Contacts and Related Subjects

The education and training of health visitors is amplified by exchanges of information with those involved in related subjects.

Reproduced by courtesy of The Nursing Times

SECTION 2 SUPPLEMENT 2

PROGRESS REPORT

In January 1978 a paper was prepared for Chairman's Committee (CC/78/8) "Planning for 1978", the detail of which is reproduced in *Column 1* of this paper.

In July 1980 a check was made on each of these items and action taken was noted. This is summarised in *Column 2:*

	Column 1	*Column 2*
A.	**Consolidation of initiatives taken in 1977-necessary sequels**	Action Taken
a.	HVT Course, Scotland	Established at Jordanhill
b.	School nursing syllabus	Published and circulated, CETHV responsibility recognised.
c.	Further education for health visitors including syllabus planning, courses for assessors of supervised practice, and the investigation into the quality of fieldwork practice.	Two Reports on Further Education.
d.	Multidisciplinary courses	Nottingham Symposium-arranged by CCETSW, Panel of Assessors, RCGP and CETHV.
e.	Curriculum development with reference to the principles and practice exercise, the Court Report and "Violence in the Family" etc.	Interim Report to Council, July 1980.
f.	Training Rules	Amended.
g.	The EEC and the public health nurse	Contact with UK representatives. Staff on EEC Study Tours.
h.	Policy on obstetrics	Specially designed courses arranged throughout UK.
i	Fieldwork teacher's certificate course.	Revised and established.
j.	Conversion course for H.V.	Planned and established.
k.	Publications, including the new handbook	Handbook published, and various publications.
l.	Open Days	Held in England, Scotland and N Ireland for Nurse Managers, DNEs etc.

m. Development of meetings with health visitor tutors	Meetings held in five centres, twice a year.
B. Proposed new developments	
a. Study of statistical basis for training programme including effect on recruitment policy	Manpower Study-first print-out 1980.
b. Statement on HVT ratios.	Modifications suggested by Education Committee.
c. Study of implications of extending the health visitor course	Receiving attention in connection with Curriculum Development.
d. Investigating the possibility of the health visitor certificate becoming a CNAA diploma	Receiving attention in connection with Curriculum Development.
e. HVT course developments	Establishment of course at University of Surrey. Development at Wolverhampton.
f. Consideration of the Establishment of an Advisory Committee for England	Arrangements under way.
g. Study days for training officers	Considered in relation to development of FE.
h. Research Committee developments, including the possibility of the establishment of a research unit.	List of priorities prepared, ½-time services of Research Officer agreed.

July 1980

SECTION 3

MAJOR DEVELOPMENTS

Stimulation for changes in established practices as well as for innovations was coming by now from external sources as well as from the Council itself. Some of the development which resulted might be considered for adoption elsewhere.

The Stimulation of Developments

It may appear invidious to select examples of major developments during the "Middle Years" without first mentioning the efforts made by Council members and staff to ensure that changes made in connection with the routine work of the Council were carried out as they became necessary. The re-design of a form, the re-shaping of the Council's records system, the plans for up-dating Regulations, or such a major exercise as the revision of the Council's "Handbook" for the use of those offering courses, were not likely to "hit the headlines", but they were nevertheless time-consuming and had to be given full attention if the smooth running of the Council's business was to continue. Undoubtedly too, the careful scrutiny of an individual's application to gain entry to the Health Visitor Tutors' Roll was of paramount importance to the person concerned. Similarly, the conditions, (if any), of the Council's approval of a Health Visitor course were of great importance to the relevant institution. Nevertheless, in terms of an historic record, it is necessary to select for special mention some of the major innovatory developments which took place during this period.

The stimuli for these developments came from a number of sources or sometimes a combination of sources. Some came as a direct result of the Strategy Exercise and sequels, which had indicated in particular that extra attention might be given especially to the functions relating to Further Education and Research. Others appeared as natural sequels to established practice, for example the system of Visitations which was added to the approvals procedure. The main impetus for the study of the "Principles of Health Visiting" (Ref 12) came from the Health Visitor Tutors who attended their Annual Conference in 1974.

By now this group as a whole had overcome many initial difficulties and had not only established itself successfully in institutions of Higher Education (six promoted to Head of Department) but had gained conspicuously from the width of experience that Universities and Colleges offered. The kind of critical analysis now produced was

(Ref 12) "An Investigation into the Principles of Health Visiting" pub CETHV 1977

thought to be exceptional for a profession at that time. The Manpower Planning Exercise (see Page 44) was stimulated by the necessity for a more substantial factual basis for decision-making on the planning of student places and was taken forward on the initiative of Research Committee members making use of their personal expertise and of facilities that they themselves could offer. Pressure for the School Nurse Syllabus came from the profession itself. The development of "Satellite" courses arose in the first place out of an immediate need to make local provision for education and training to match the recruitment drive started by an employer following an enquiry into a case of child neglect. This scheme added extra places for students within a locality as a short-term measure without committing educational resources long-term. Many changes too were influenced by a number of indications coming together from different sources, the evidence from the Professional Advisers' visits to the Managers and to the Educational Institutions, the comments made to the author at the meetings of Tutors, the knowledge gained from a variety of groups met on Visitations' and, not least, the experience and considerations of Council members themselves. Added to this, the Council now found itself required to respond to proposals for developments taking place within educational institutions which might involve Health Visitors. Examples of the many initiatives now occurring were : 1. the BA Education course at Wolverhampton College, which might allow entry to prospective Health Visitor Tutor students if the plans were agreed by Council and 2. the development of the Health Studies courses in Queen Margaret College Edinburgh and Glasgow College of Technology - the former "Diploma in Life Science/Nursing" and the latter "Diploma in Nursing Studies" later to be translated into Degree Courses. Other developments ranged from the University of Manchester to the South Bank Polytechnic and from Milton Keynes to the Polytechnic of Ulster. The story was one of continuing movement and apart from the very serious setback in recruitment during this period, it would be difficult to find any area of the Council's responsiblities where it would not be claimed that considerable developments had taken place during the "Middle Years".

Further Education

A comprehensive plan for "Continuing Education" for Health Visitors was the subject of two Council reports, in 1977 and 1980. The first (Ref 13) included the results of questionnaires and letters to practising Health Visitors and Service Managers and resulted in the design of a flow-chart which suggested further education and

(Ref 13) Preliminary 'Report of a Working Group on Further Education'. 1977

training developments for Health Visitors in terms of vertical and lateral growth (see Section 3 Supplement 1). This report also offered aims and objectives for a variety of educational and training activities. In the summary it is stated that "progressive staff development linked with Performance Review, is a cornerstone in the development of a competent practising Health Visitor, and therefore a basic course of education and training should be followed by a variety of on-going special skills courses, such as Developmental Paediatrics and Hearing Testing, and specific subject courses such as Counselling and Mental Health." It adds "There is a lack of any overall policy on identification of needs both at national and local level. Co-ordination and control of further education and training policies in relation to national needs and more effective co-ordination and co-operation is required."

The second report (Ref 14) had within its terms of reference "To provide a progressive pattern of personal and professional development leading to increasing competence in various aspects of health visiting; and to make recommendations as to the methods by which this can be done." The eventual suggestions made included the establishment of two categories of further education courses for Health Visitors, namely "Recognised Courses" and "Courses suitable for Health Visitors" and proposed the establishment of "Further Education Liaison Groups" including representatives both from Education and Service. It was suggested further that Council should give priority to the consideration of "Recognised Courses" in the first instance and subsequently to the "Suitable Courses." This was seen as "fundamental to any cost-effective planning." This report was circulated for comment in December 1980. Between them these two reports offered the comprehensive programme of Continuing Education: the first indicated the extent and variety of courses required and the second a plan aimed at ensuring further the quality of the provision.

Courses for Health Visitor Tutors, Fieldwork Teachers and Assessors of Supervised Practice.

In the first "The History of the Council" reference was made to Health Visitor Tutor courses and the fact that the Council took over the responsiblity for maintaining the Roll of Health Visitor Tutors from the Royal College of Nursing in 1967. During the "Middle Years" the centres for Health Visitor Tutor courses changed from the two centres at the Royal College and at Bolton College of Education to the pattern of two "major" centres now to be at the University of

(Ref 14) "Handbook of Further Education for Health Visitors," 1980

Surrey and at Bolton and the additional facilities for meeting small local demands at Wolverhampton College and at Jordanhill in Glasgow. Special provision was made also for two other groups: the first, for graduate Health Visitors undertaking the M.Sc Nurse Tutor course at Edinburgh Univeristy to follow on with the appropriate additions to qualify as eligible for the Health Visitor Tutor Roll; the second for qualified teachers who also had the required Health Visiting experience to undertake a specially-designed "Conversion" course.

All those who have visited Health Visitor courses are left in no doubt that the influence and ability of Health Visitor Tutors is of prime importance and, therefore, all decisions on the suitability of course provision for Tutors were only taken after extensive deliberation. First of all, there was the problem of small numbers. If, say, about 30 Health Visitor Tutors a year were to qualify, the number of centres must be limited in order to ensure groups of an effective size. At the same time, the call for local provision was becoming louder as the ratio of married women with home commitments increased. But to give way to this call and allow student Health Visitor Tutors to be attached, say, to all Nurse Tutor courses in ones and twos (a group who in any case are being prepared for teaching mainly in monotechnic establishments, within the Health as opposed to the Education Service) might provide an extra element in the Nurse Tutor course but could dilute the specialist interest of Health Visitor Tutors to an unacceptable degree. The reasoning behind the Council's early decision to site courses in Universities and Polytechnics were explained in the first History of the CETHV and now the Council's insistence that HVT courses should be placed alongside those of other F.E. Teachers can be understood as a logical sequel to the early decisions. This philosophy was included in the thinking that lay behind Council's decision not to recognise the RCN's proposal for the New University of London Diploma in Nursing Education course, as suitable for the preparation of Health Visitors Tutors, while placing on record its gratitude to the College for pioneering the original Health Visitor Tutor course in 1948. The long-standing problem of central funding for Health Visitor Tutors and selection was raised again in connection with discussions in the Briggs Co-ordinating Committee (Working Group 3) and resulted in the recommendation that central funding should be established for Health Visitor Tutors (as well as District Nurse Tutors and Midwife Teachers) and included the phrase "Generally speaking, the CETHV could operate a scheme in which the Council was allocated funds by the Government Departments and would then reimburse the seconding Authority."

Fieldwork Teachers Courses

As at least one third of the HV Course is followed in the practical field, the Council from the first recognised the importance of the Instructor/Teacher and encouraged extra preparation for this role. The early development of first Fieldwork Instructor courses, later Fieldwork Teacher courses, was described in the first "History". This development continued during the "Middle Years" and in 1979 a revised syllabus giving guidance and regulations for a Certificate course in Fieldwork Teaching was passed by Council. It contained the plans for a course divided into two parts, Part I taken in the first year normally containing six weeks full-time study on a block release basis and Part II taken in the second year consisting of practice under supervision; the 2 parts together offering these practising HVs the opportunity to study a wider base of relevant knowledge and, in particular, further study of teaching skills. In planning for this development of the Fieldwork Teachers course, it had been recognised by the Working Party that every effort must be made to have regard to the financial constraints of the day. Nevertheless, it was felt possible to offer a new type of syllabus based on an analysis of the work of the Fieldwork Teacher and which included for the first time a method for withdrawal if an individual was considered unsuitable for this particular work at the end of Part I. This course would in any case be of use to the HV, as 'further education'. It also included the requirement of supervision during the second year before a certificate was granted. This provision virtually intensified and made as an official requirement the usual custom of the Health Visitor Tutor offering guidance to the Fieldwork Teacher during her first year of practice.

The implementation, however, was not accomplished without some difficulties. There were some complaints from Service Managers that insufficient consultation had taken place, from College Tutors who became aware of the extra work involved and from some College Administrators who found themselves with some problems in relation to a course where Part I and Part II might be undertaken in different establishments. These administrative difficulties were taken to a meeting held at Clifton House and were talked out between those who had found solutions to the problems and those whose particular problems remained unresolved at that time. While time alone will show more clearly the merits or de-merits of this new plan, initial reactions to the course itself suggested that both Health Visitor Tutors and Fieldwork Teacher students found it had considerable merit. However, the apparently intractable problem of the Fieldwork Teacher salary, (which by then had to be considered alongside those of Clinical Teachers as well as the Practical Work Teachers) remained as a constant threat to the continuation of the arrangements for the Health Visitor students' practical work.

Assessors of Supervised Practice Courses

In addition to responsibilities given to the Health Visitor Tutors and Fieldwork Teachers, the role of the Assessor of Supervised Practice at the end of the Health Visitor course was clearly of paramount importance. It was not surprising, therefore, that the need for some form of preparation had become apparent and initiative had been taken in a number of centres in establishing short courses of two of five days duration for these Assessors. In January 1978, a Working Group met to "consider the role and function of the Assessors of the student Health Visitor during the period of supervised practice and the preparations needed to undertake their task." The final recommendations were passed on to Council from Professional Development Committee and included the suggestion that courses should be established based on the outline given, of not less than five days duration taken either on a full or equivalent part-time basis, these courses to be "approved" by Council. For this exercise, a more elaborate system of early consultation was set up. The results showed a wide diversity of views among Service Managers but there was sufficent support by the majority for the Council to proceed.

Courses in School Nursing.

It had become a matter of increasing concern to Health Visitors that the School Nurses with whom they worked were under-prepared. The possibility of developing a syllabus for School Nurses was first mentioned at a Council meeting in 1975, but it was not until 1977, following correspondence with the DHSS, that the Council found itself in a position to offer the first CETHV "Guidelines to a Syllabus for a Course in School Nursing" and later to be able to receive applications for the approval of courses and formally record the names of successful candidates. The proposals were for a three-month course with two months theory and one of practice to be organised in institutions where there were Health Visitor Courses already established. The report included aims and objectives, qualifications for entry, duration of course, subjects for a syllabus and practical training etc. It stated that some difficulty had been experienced in so far as "a definite role for the school nurse" has yet to be given by the Government Departments. In view of the Council's legal position, exceptional care was taken to ensure that all parties were aware of the situation. However, the Council had reason to be reassured further in so far as official encouragement was given later for it to continue this work by designing a course for nurses caring for the physically handicapped child. This exercise was then carrried out resulting in a course specially designed to follow on from the basic course in School Nursing for this particular group. However, it was realised that as the number of potential students was relatively small, it would only be practicable to offer such a course on a regional/national basis, if and when application for approval of such a course should be received. By the end of 1980, a number of courses in School Nursing had received Council's approval including the first application from Scotland where planning had been postponed while the results of a specific study in School Nursing were considered.

Curriculum Development

In January 1978 a Working Party of Education Committee was set up to advise on the subject of Curriculum Development, but it soon became apparent that a wider representation was required and a newly constituted Working Party composed of representatives of all the main Committees of the Council took over the task in May 1979. Early stages of the work included the production of a plan of progression, collection of evidence on job descriptions of health visiting staff and the study of "behavioural objectives" taken at two working conferences of Health Visitor Tutors in 1978/79. Alongside this activity was an "Investigation into the principles of Health Visiting" which was carried out by a group composed mainly of Health Visitor Tutors with the support of Council's staff, working to the terms of reference prescribed by Education Committee but allowing the group maximum independence and freedom of action within those terms. This searching investigation had explored the principles of Health Visiting in the first instance to ensure the validity of the teaching. This in itself provided a lead into the study of Curriculum Development which was to make a critical appraisal of the syllabus of the Health Visitor Course in order to ensure the precise preparation required by this profession for work in the 1980s. The early stages of the Working Party on Curriculum Development were not without difficulty, not least because of unavoidable changes in membership. And again, history was to repeat itself as the Working Party found, as had been found by its predecessors in 1963, that it was necessary first to study in detail the present role of the Health Visitor. Only when this had been done on the basis of the analysis of quantities of documentary evidence, could the study of Curriculum Development as such really begin. The report to Council in June 1979 stated that decisions had been made regarding operational definition of terms, terms of reference, a programme of activities for the Working Party, and a time schedule for the completion of the programme. As the subject of Curriculum Development was central to the future of Health Visitor Education and Training, and required a complexity of studies and consultations, this searching exercise was unlikely to be completed for some time.

Health Visitor Manpower Investigation

Following "pilot investigations" and discussions with the statistics branches of the Health Departments, the Council decided to undertake a comprehensive enquiry throughout the United Kingdom, to be up-dated annually, which would not only enable the Council to assess with much greater precision than at present the probable future requirements for student Health Visitor places, but would also provide for the first time the major part of a register of practising Health Visitors. Additionally, it would enable statistical information to be given to Health Authorities about future manpower projections, which because of the comprehensiveness of the data, would be statistically more reliable than information derived from within one Area or Board (or Region) alone. In the past, care had been taken to bring in to focus all known facts before a new centre for a Health Visitor course was established. The information available, however, did not include such data as the average duration of a Health Visitor's career, or the frequency of changes of post due to promotion, which in itself would have an effect on potential demand for student places. Results of pilot schemes, for example, had indicated that possibly 25% of Health Visitors went on to work in either an administrative or teaching post. The Chairman of Research Committee, himself Chairman of an Area Health Authority and Head of a University Social Science Department, was able to offer computer facilities and the first attempt to obtain returns was made in 1979. The returns were not as comprehensive as hoped, but the material was sufficient to allow for the production of computerised results for some parts of the United Kingdom. Some reluctance in completing returns arose over questions of confidentiality, for although the Council had specifically said that it would be glad to receive notice of difficulties and offer further advice, this message appeared not to have penetrated "down the line." However, the results of this first analysis were fed back for the information of those Authorities who had completed the questionnaires and a 'mock' return was supplied for the interest of the Authorities who had not responded on the first round. The most useful results could only be obtained in the long term if returns reach 100%, but even on a more limited sample a picture of trends was beginning to build up. In spite of some imperfections, this proved to be an innovatory exercise which could provide a 'tool' to decision making never before available. In view of this Council's statutory responsibilities and Research Committee's new initiatives, it was particularly disappointing that this particular Statutory Body still awaited permission to appoint a Research Worker to the staff.

Other Developments

The Council noted in several instances developments in Higher and Further Education which could have application to the work of the Council. Certainly, the idea of a 'Satelite' course bore some resemblance to the established pattern in Management courses where 'centres of excellence' had been established, mainly in Polytechnics, which supplied staff with expertise to other Colleges. The pattern of 'Visitations' had some resemblance in a very abbreviated form to the practices of the Council for National Academic Awards. In the case of the CETHV, a team composed of members of Council and members of staff was organised in the first instance to visit the Institution when the "Confirmatory Review" was required for newly established courses and later included courses of long standing applying for re-approval. During these exercises, every care was taken to try and ensure that the staff of the Institution would feel free to exchange views with the visiting party and that a mutually informative and constructive exercise would result. With the visiting party working to a self-imposed "code", the overall conclusions appeared to have been firstly that the Education Committee of the Council was able now to base its decisions on a fuller understanding of the applications than had been possible before and, secondly, that the visit by a team from Council provided the occasion for Council's business to be taken to the highest level in the institution concerned. These visits, however, for practical reasons could be conducted only on the limited scale of approximately five per year. Other approvals continued to be considered on the basis of data supplied by the institution supplemented by the Professional Adviser's knowledge of the establishment and the personal appearance of the Tutor in charge at the Committee meeting if he/she wished. During the "Middle Years," the variety of courses for which Council approval was required had developed and now not only the basic course but Fieldwork Teachers and Assessors of Supervised Practice and the courses for School Nurses had been added. This situation, coupled with the fact that the institutions themselves had acquired considerable expertise in this area of work, raised the question as to whether the time had come for a different approval procedure to be considered.

The Council files reveal that developments have depended upon the opportunities offered within the Health and the Education Services, the availability of resources and, not least, the human element, for without the hard work, the persistence and at least a touch of imaginative thinking on the part of those involved in the planning, none of these advances would ever have taken place.

SECTION 3 SUPPLEMENT 1

Council for the Education and Training of Health Visitors
Clifton House, Euston Road, London NW1 2RS Telephone 01 387 3456

SUGGESTED FURTHER EDUCATION & TRAINING DEVELOPMENT FOR HEALTH VISITORS

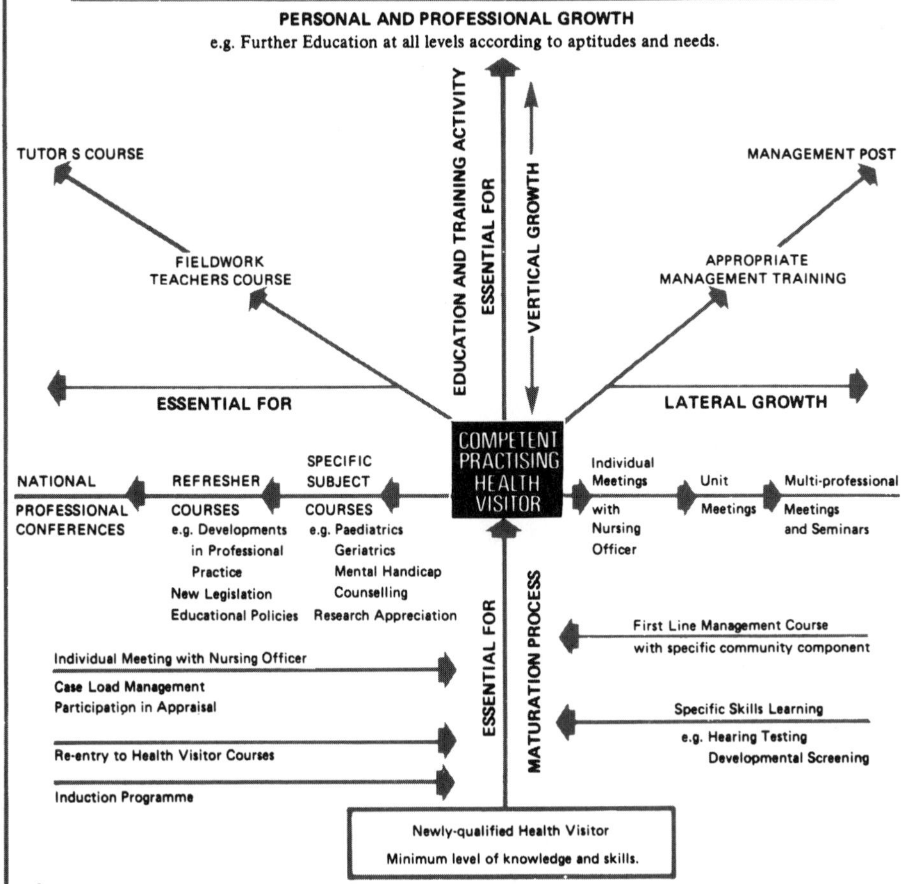

✱ Suggested Flow Chart for Further Education and Training of Health Visitors.

SECTION 4

THE ROLE OF A U.K. STATUTORY BODY

At this time, the C.E.T.H.V. was the only Statutory Body in this field with responsibilities covering the whole of the U.K. The Council's National Advisory Committees had been established at different time and had chosen to operate in a variety of ways. While these differences had to be respected, powers were retained centrally by the Council, thus providing a means of establishing some uniformity of standards in courses and the added advantage in such a comparatively small profession of the interchange of information and ideas across national boundaries. The Council's international links were developed further as Health Departments in many other parts of the world were concentrating increasing attention and resources on 'prevention' and on 'primary care'.

The Establishment of the Four National Advisory Committees

Before any worthwhile account can be given of the Council's role as a U.K. Statutory Body, it is necessary to describe briefly the history of the establishment of the four National Advisory Committees, their individual features and some indication of the way in which they relate to the Council itself.

Reference was made in Sections 1 and 2 to the establishment of the Scottish Advisory Committee and the Northern Ireland Advisory Committee and the later establishment of the Welsh Advisory Committee in 1975 and the English Advisory Committee in 1980. The reasons for this apparently illogical development were, in the first instance, the wording of the 1962 Act which mentioned the Scottish Advisory Committee and the Northern Ireland Advisory Committee, which were to be serviced by the Health Departments of those countries, but omitted reference to England and Wales. By 1975, however, with the establishment of a third centre in Wales, there seemed to the Council to be reasons enough to give Wales a similar facility and this was done by appointing like representatives to a Welsh Advisory Committee, the servicing of this Committee to be carried out by Council staff. The possibility of the establishment of an English Advisory Committee had been raised a number of times over the years but, while the idea had been championed continually by some members of Council, it had failed to gain the unanimous support of Council until 1980. No doubt this reluctance was due to some extent to the very heavy commitment to Council's business placed upon members by the combined demands for extensive developments and now the extra calls arising out of the proposals for the 1979 Act. In retrospect, there seems to be little reason for the illusion, and illusion it proved to be, that a London-based Council was preoccupied with English matters. A detailed analysis had revealed that apart from the advantage of ease of access to meetings at the headquarters, England was "missing out" on such matters as the study of the problems of local recruitment. Further stimulation was provided by the realisation that under the 1979 Act all four countries were to have National Boards which in turn would be required to communicate with the Health Visiting Joint Committee on all matters relating to Health Visiting (Ref 15).

The Advisory Committees displayed different features which in some ways related to their settings. The Scottish Advisory Committee, the longest established Committee and, until 1980, the Committee concerned with the interests of the largest country, had the most wide-ranging discussions. It had instigated a number of studies on topics of particular national interest such as the "triple duty nurse," the "unqualified Health Visitor", "recruitment" and in dealing with the request from the GNC in Scotland on comments on 'Future Schemes for Student Nurse Training in Scotland' (1977). It was from Scotland, too, that pressure came for an immediate statement on the relationship between the Health Visitor and the new District Nursing courses. The Northern Ireland Advisory Committee had been interested to receive an annual account of the progress and recruitment and other developments at their one training centre and of the progress towards the establishment of a second centre which eventually occurred in 1980. In the intimate atmosphere of the Province, it was not unusual for topics relating to the service to be raised. It appeared that the Health Visiting profession here felt exceptionally threatened by the Health and Personal Social Services Order 1972 and at meetings of the Advisory Committee the opportunity was sometimes taken to raise general issues. This, however, was outside the remit of the Council's business and could be taken no further. It was interesting to note, nevertheless, that following some discussions which had started within the Advisory Committee, a liaison group between Health Visitors and General Practitioners became established. Again, arising out of particular local pressures, a plan was initiated by the Advisory Committee and taken up by Ulster Polytechnic for the production of video-tapes on Health Visiting for the use of various student groups with the purpose of relieving the load on practising Health Visitors. The Welsh Advisory Committee opted from the start for a half-day session with a

(Ref 15) Nurses, Midwives and Health Visitors Act 1979. Section 8

speaker in the morning, followed by a half-day session on Council business. It obtained from Council permission to extend the original membership so as to include a representative from each course, and each AHA in Wales, a provision which was practicable in a country the size of Wales. This Advisory Committee also agreed to vary the location of their meetings, including the provision that one meeting a year should be in the north of Wales. Topics taken by the Welsh Advisory Committee included a survey of applications for Health Visitor places and consideration on the future of the Welsh Advisory Committee following the passing of the 1979 Act. At all Advisory Committee meetings the minutes of Council meetings were made available and were discussed. All Advisory Committees, too, were involved in the preparation of Council 'Comments' in so far as they concerned the individual country.

It was not possible to gauge to what extent the activities of one Advisory Committee had direct repercussions in another, but there is substantial evidence to prove that matters first raised in an Advisory Committee, such as the relationship between the District Nurse and Health Visitors courses, influenced ultimately the actions of the Council and thus have affected the whole.

The U.K. Commitment

The U.K. commitment, it has proved, brought a wide range of responsibilities, opportunities and practical demands. Perhaps it can be taken as some measure of the success with which the Council has tackled the tasks that wishes were expressed from all quarters during the Devolution Debate (see Section 1) that the education and training of Health Visitors should remain in the hands of a U.K. body. This conclusion appeared to have been founded on the recognition of two potentially opposing factors: first the very real differences between the four countries of the United Kingdom and, secondly, the recognition of what is the same in terms of the Council's business.

Differences which had to be given due consideration included cultural patterns, geographical features, legal provision, the policies of the Health and Education services and the development of the related professions. And finally there was the very important factor of difference in size as illustrated by the number of training centres: 37 in England, 6 in Scotland, 3 in Wales and 2 in Northern Ireland. Size, too, might partially account for the fact that the Chief Nursing Officer herself in Northern Ireland had attended Advisory Committee meetings when possible, thus becoming the first and to date the only Chief Nursing Officer to gain personal experience of the business meetings of this particular Statutory Body.

Both in terms of common courtesy and of political expediency, respect for the differences in the four countries was essential and while each country had its own Health Department and Education Department, a U.K. body had to have regard for four (or eight) "masters". In negotiating with all the other Statutory Bodies, it had been necessary also to appreciate considerable national differences; for example, the standard of entry to Nurse Training in England and in Scotland respectively.

The Council had been aware also of a wide variation in the degree of interest shown in the development of Health Visiting. While some of those in senior posts following the reorganisation of the National Health Service were convinced of the importance of a preventive service, whether Health Visiting was in their own range of experience or not, others who were fully committed to the interests of Nursing and Midwifery continued to see the interests of Health Visiting to be of secondary significance. All these variables were important and had to be remembered in one way or another while the Council attempted to fulfill the legal obligations placed upon it.

As well as the differences, it was, of course, necessary to consider the similarities or common factors. This immediately raised the question of the basic skills of the Health Visiting profession, for only when this was established could the Health Visitor course be planned, albeit in the knowledge that it would be necessary to adapt the use of these skills to variations in the fields of practice in these islands, and indeed to conditions in other corners of the world.

Particular Features of a U.K. Organisation

The activities of the Council during the "Middle Years" suggest the particular features of a U.K. organisation include the following:-

1. Council meetings-
   (a) should be held in Scotland, Northern Ireland and Wales as well as England;
   (b) reports of National Advisory Committees should be given high priority on the Council's agenda;
2. Membership of Council's main Committees;-
   should be formed as far as possible from a cross-section of representatives from all four countries.
3. Communications - must be retained with :-
   (a) Health Departments and Education Departments (all countries). NB - it is especially important that legal matters should be referred to all Departments concerned;
   (b) related Professional Organisations (all countries):
   (c) related Statutory and non-Statutory Bodies (all countries);
   (d) Service Managers (all countries).

4. National Advisory Committee Meetings -
   (a) must be attended by the assigned Professional Adviser to that country and the Council's Chief Officers;
   (b) "comments" on matters pertaining to an individual country must be prepared by and agreed by the Advisory Committee from Council;
   (c) the agenda must contain items particular to the country concerned as well as the Council's business as a whole.
5. Individual Arrangements:-
   (a) separate negotiations will be required where different national bodies are involved, e.g. midwifery;
   (b) ad hoc meetings may be necessary where particular national problems arise;
   (c) discussion on new proposals, e.g. the Reports on Further Education, must be in terms of England, Wales, Scotland and Northern Ireland.
6. Publications and Circulated Information-
   must be distributed to all Authorities equally throughout the United Kingdom.
7. Staffing -
   In the case of Scotland, Northern Ireland and Wales, one Professional Adviser to be assigned for each as first contact between the Council and the Educational Institutions and the Service Managers in each country. Each Professional Adviser concerned must also carry an assignment outside the boundaries of that country to assist in the cross-fertilization of ideas (in the case of England, the Professional Adviser's assignment was designed to correspond very approximately with one or more Regional boundaries). While the assigned Professional Adviser was the first contact, all specialist knowledge must be available as need arises, as well as the services of the senior members of staff.
8. General considerations -
   The workload of a Statutory Body which is required to carry out functions on a U.K. basis is considerably greater than would be required for a similar assignment on a national basis only. This needs to be reflected in the number of members as well as the numbers of staff.

International Affairs

International links continued to grow during this period. Visitors were received in the Council's office as individuals and in groups and members of staff travelled overseas. These experiences revealed a widespread interest in prevention and community care in both advanced and developing countries. Therefore, while those with interests in Health Visiting may have reasons on occasions to feel that they are "prophets without honour in their own country", the Council has been left in no doubt of the interest in preventive services overseas. This contrast in attitudes was particularly evident at the ICN Congress in Tokyo in 1977 where many representatives from different countries were speaking on the importance of the preventive services, but the U.K. representatives, nominated by the RCN, were offering papers on aspects of institutional care alone. On the basis of the evidence of international interests gained from many quarters, the Council proposed in 1979 that consideration should be given to the possibility of mounting an International Conference concerned with the provision of Public Health Nursing and the education and training of the persons involved.

Public Relations

Attempts have been made throughout the history of the Council to be mindful of public relations by means of personal contact, meetings, conferences, films and publications. In the "Middle Years." this work was increased vastly as a by-product of the Reorganisation of the National Health Service. As far as internal arrangements were concerned, it was decided eventually that Education Committee should have an oversight of publications, with an in-house group of members of the professional and the administrative staff considering the necessary on-going routine work regarding the issue of pamphlets etc. The Council's first film was replaced by "One Step Ahead" in 1979 and the twice-a-year publication of the Bulletin became more formalised. In all, three more books were published under the auspices of the Council, making a total of four (see Section 4, Supplement 1).

An unexpected boost to the Council's public relations came as a by-product of the activities in relation to the passage of the 1979 Act. Specially prepared papers were sent to all MPs, which were quoted in Parliament on occasions, and further material was sent to the House of Lords. Added to this was the responsible and effective lobbying by Health Visitors themselves which left recipients in little doubt about the activities of the Council in the past and the concern that this kind of provision should continue in the future.

SECTION 4 SUPPLEMENT 1

CETHV PUBLICATIONS

The Work of the Nursing Team in General Practice
An Investigation into the Principles of Health Visiting
The History of the Council for the Education and Training of Health Visitors.
The Investigation Debate

CETHV Films

"Quite an Education" 1979
"Live and Learn" 1973
"One step ahead" 1979

SECTION 5

THE PASSAGE OF THE 1979 ACT

In 1970 the Government set up a committee under the Chairmanship of Professor Asa Briggs (later Lord Briggs) "to review the role of nurses and midwives in the hospital and the community and the education and training required for that role".

The main recommendations of the subsequent "Report of the Committee on Nursing" included the following:-

- *i* *That there should be a single central body for professional standards, education and discipline in nursing and midwifery in Great Britain.*
- *ii* *That the responsibility for education should remain with the Department of Health.*
- *iii* *That education should be arranged as a continuing process under unified control.*
- *iv* *That colleges of nursing and midwifery should be set up.*

Following publication of this Report, interested organisations including the Council were invited to submit comments and in the case of the Council the response indicated considerable disappointment.

In subsequent years, however, the Chief Officers of the relevant existing Statutory and Non-Statutory Bodies met at intervals and discussed the practical implications of the Report in a constructive manner, first informally and then formally, at the Department of Health. But it was not until 1976 that the Secretary of State called a meeting of representatives of these bodies and of the professional organisations and unions to explore the possibility of drawing up plans for legislation arising out of the Report, which by now had become known as the "Briggs Report". A "Co-ordinating Committee", chaired by the Minister of State was established finally in January 1977 with the remit of making preparations for legislation and it concluded its meetings during the time of the final passage of the Bill in the House of Lords in the Spring of 1979.

The "Middle Years" included the latter stages of the meetings of the Chief Officers, the period of the meetings of the Co-ordinating Committee and the first pronouncements by the Government Departments regarding the implementation of the Nurses, Midwives and Health Visitors Act 1979.

From the Council's Point of View

The complete history of the passage of the 1979 Act could be compiled only after reference to the records of the many organisations involved of which the brief notes of meetings held at the DHSS and the records of events in Parliament would form only a small part. Papers held by the Council up to the end of 1980 alone extended from evidence prepared for the use of the Briggs Committee; comments on the Report of the Committee on Nursing; minutes of Council meetings and of the Council's Working Groups; correspondence with the officers of DHSS, the Minister of State (Health), MPs and members of the House of Lords; notes of meetings with MPs of all parties and documents prepared for their use. The material that follows has been selected to indicate the views of Council, the position in which it was placed by the alteration of plans and something of the atmosphere of the times.

It will be appreciated that the Council had from the time of the Report onwards remained consistent in stating and pursuing the two-fold policy of offering cooperation with Nurses and Midwives and, at the same time, requiring to be assured that the future education and training of Health Visitors was to be safeguarded. The action described, therefore, should be understood in terms of the pursuit of those policies.

The "Middle Years" saw the final preprations for and the eventual passing of the Nurses, Midwives and Health Visitors Act 1979 which was to replace previous enactments relating to all the Statutory Bodies concerned with Nursing, Midwifery and Health Visitor education and training throughout the U.K. and was to incorporate also the work of the related non-Statutory Bodies.

From the Council's viewpoint these were times when hopes and fears about the future ebbed and flowed. At times it appeared that provision was to be made within the proposed Act for Health Visitor education and training to be continued on a U.K. basis on the lines the Council had worked so hard to establish, only to find these hopes dashed by the powerful forces of larger organisations. In the event, Council's views, which had claimed so little of the attention, it appeared, on the original Briggs Committee, continued largely to be ignored by the Health Departments and by the Minister's "Co-ordinating Committee" set up in 1977 to prepare the ground for the new legislation. With the future provision for Health Visitor education seemingly imperilled, the Council's appeal for consideration was carried forward to MPs and members of the House of Lords as the Bill progressed. This responsible 'lobbying' by the Council, also by organisations such as the HVA, the Standing

Conference of HV Training Centres and the Committee of Directors of Polytechnics and, not least, by individual Health Visitors themselves received a sympathetic hearing and - as Hansard records - had a marked effect on the Parliamentary debates.

The wording of the clause to be included concerning the eastablishment of a 'Joint Committee' for Health Visitors (and possibly for other groups) became the major area of dispute M.P.s themselves expressing surprise that this Bill had been put forward as 'non-controversial'. Finally, it was promised that a newly worded clause would be added to the Bill when it reached the Lords if the bodies concerned could produce an agreed alternative. The point had been reached by this time when some were questioning the future of the Bill itself and then, and only then, a compromise form of words was found and agreed by the Co-ordinating Committee and the passage of the Bill move forward.

This clause was to allow for the establishment of a Health Visitor Joint Committee which had to be consulted on all matters relating to Health Visiting; with permissive powers only for function to be delegated by the United Kingdom Central Council or the National Board now to be established to this Committee. Thus the CETHV was to hand over the comprehensive legal powers it had deployed with some effect for 20 years to the less clearly defined responsibilities of the UKCC, the National Boards and the Joint Committee.

'Extract from the Council's Papers (Supplement 1) records the most significant stages in the passage of the 1979 Act. First there were the hopeful signs in 1975 and the spring of 1976 when it was reported that the principle of a Health Visitor Joint Committee for Health Visitors with legal powers was to be established within the proposed Bill. This position, however, was then significantly eroded by the suggestions put forward in the Health Department's paper 'The Statutory Framework' and "Briggs further action" circulated in the name of the Chief Nursing Officer in February 1977. The Council made clear its disagreement with these much modified proposals. Nevertheless, in the Press Release which followed the first meeting of the "Co-ordinating Committee" under the Chairmanship of the Minister of State (Health) it was stated that 'There was a broad measure of agreement - a few areas needed further discussion'. By September 1977, the Author wrote to the Council's Chairman "what the Council had believed to be re-assurances on the future for Health Visitor education and training was no longer part of the plan". Following a meeting of Council's representatives with the Minister of State, however, fears were allayed by his personal assurance that the "the whole purpose of establishing a Statutory Health Visitor

Committee was to retain the present pattern of Health Visitor Education''.

Resistance to the concept of such a Statutory (Joint) Committee for Health Visitors as well as some special provision for Midwifery was voiced by a number of other specialist groups e.g. Psychiatric Nurses and others, for example, the influential RCN representative continued to voice objections. Later, however, the RCN voice was modified when its District Nurse and Health Visitor members asked that their views also should be given consideration. The question of Statutory Committees, with or without 'powers' remained the central point of controversy throughout.

In July 1978, the author was asked by Council to raise the possibility of an alternative plan for a 'Federation', a plan which later received the official support of the Central Midwives Board but was rejected by the representatives of other organisations. In October 1978, Council's Chairman wrote to the Minister asking if he would consider ''publishing a White or perhaps a Green Paper setting out the case for change and the Government's proposals'' - again without result. At the meeting of Council on October 19th, the DHSS representative made it clear that the CETHV could not 'opt out' of the new legislation and the Council's attention then moved to making representations to Parliament.

In November 1978, the Council's hopes were raised again when an invitation was received to meet the Minister following a productive meeting he had had with the Midwives organisations. After some delays and apparent significant internal negotiations, the Minister eventually stated he was not prepared to offer any amendments himself to meet the CETHV requests.

The subsequent period, while the Bill passed through the various stages in Parliament was not without some consolation to the Council. A great deal of sympathy was expressed for the Council's viewpoint as well as praise for the work it had done and for the efforts of Health Visitors themselves. The final struggle to find a form of words for Clause 8 (Joint Committee) acceptable to all parties was left to the Co-ordinating Committee members and, with the possibility now of the withdrawal of support for the Bill, a compromise was reached. The wording which was added to the Bill when it reached the House of Lords made it obligatory for the Central Council and National Boards to refer matters relating to Health Visiting to 'their' Joint Committee and made it possible for legal functions to be allocated to it. This compromise position, however, represented a considerable concession on the part of the Council and left the future of Health Visitor education and training in a vulnerable position.

In July 1979, the Council was informed that the new (Conservative) Minister of State (Health) was considering the question of delaying the implementation of the new Act. Before Council had met and had had the opportunity to respond to the letter, however, a second letter was received stating that the Minister had been left in no doubt by the reactions received to his first letter and implementation was to be set underway by an Order to be laid in Parliament. A subsequent request that the Council might act as 'Shadow' Health Visitor Joint Committee was turned down.

The supplements illustrate these events as follows:-

Supplement 1 "Extracts for Council's Paper" = quotations from Council Meeting Minutes etc.

Supplement 2 An example of the 'Record of Events' = a paper prepared for Council Meeting March 1979 illustrating the extent of action taken.

Supplement 3 'Articles and Papers relating to the Briggs Legislation' = a list of printed material and booklets for the use of MPs.

Supplement 4 'Quotations from the Press'.

Supplement 5 'The Authors analysis of related influences and events' = a selection of facts and impressions by one who was witness to these events.

SECTION 5 SUPPLEMENT 1

(a) *Extracts from Council Papers*

2 March 1975 Matters arising out of the Minutes of Council Meeting 22 January.

'The Director's report on the final discussion in which she and *Miss Fraser (Council Member) had participated with* Government Departments and other Statutory Bodies on 26 February, the proposals were generally welcomed as allaying many of the fears expressed by Council in the past, and the proposal that the Statutory Health Visiting Committee would be a central body with continuing responsibility for the U.K. was especially welcome.''

(This was the final report from the first Director of Council)

[During 1975 informal meetings continued to take place among groups of Chief Officers - these meetings superseded by the ''Joint Liaison Committee'' set up by the DHSS in 1976, and the meetings thereafter were called by the Health Departments ''to consider preliminary steps to be taken to facilitate the implementation of the Briggs Report.'']

March 1976 Minutes of Council Meeting. The Director reported:

''The Department accepted that the training of Health Visitors should continue to be based in the public sector'' (of education) ''and the need for a Statutory Committee had been established.''

July 1976 Council's comments on the U.K. Health Departments' paper ''The Statutory Framework''.

''The Council agrees that the statutory Health Visitor Committee should exercise delegated powers in relation to the functions of the Central Council...Council'' (the CETHV) ''is convinced that several of the functions in paragraph 7 on functions of the National Board must be exercised centrally by the statutory Health Visitor Committee of the Central Council. The Council would point out that it would not be possible for the respective National Boards to build up sufficient experience and expertise to maintain and validate properly with such small numbers ... Council wishes to express grave concern at the very significant change of authority outlined in the new document.''

[In November 1976 there was a Press Release from the Health Department announcing the Government's firm commitment to introducing the main recommendations of the Briggs Committee - followed in January 1977 by the Minister of State announcing the establishment of the Co-ordinating Committee. The first meeting of the Co-ordinating Committee took place on 20 March 1977 and, as a sequel, a letter was sent to Committee Members by the CNO (DHSS) dated 21 January on behalf of all CNOs of the U.K. inviting comments on a Paper entitled "Briggs Further Action".]

24 February 1977 Letter from Director to CNO (DHSS) in response to the paper "Briggs Further Action" after corresponding with all Council Members and agreed by Council's Chairman.

"Members of Council have asked me to reply to your letter of 21 January as follows:—

1. The study of the functions of the Central Council and the National Boards as now required, without a concurrent study of the functions of the two statutory committees is unrealistic and would lay the whole question of the education and training of health visitors open to take-over by those with inadequate knowledge or experience in this area of work.

2. The argument that the education and training should remain the responsibility of one U.K. body (or Statutory Committee) has been supported by our national advisory committees and is known to have support both in education and service quarters. This argument has been accepted already by the DHSS and has been written into previous Government documents. At a time when the Government is calling for the expansion of the health visitor service, any such move could be catastrophic."

(*17 March 1977* Press release from DHSS - "Mr. Moyle launches Briggs Working Groups"

"Mr. Moyle (Minister of State) has announced that a broad measure of agreement was reached on the main form of future legislation. There are a few areas which need further discussion.")

29 September 1977 Letter from Director to Chairman.

"At the meeting today of the full Co-ordinating Committee under Mr. Moyles's Chairmanship I have become very disturbed at the turn of events. Membership of the various Statutory Committees was discussed ... in terms of feasibility for individual members who might be required to attend business for the Central Council, National Board and Statutory Committee- it simply does not work.

"And a second onslaught on our interests was the implication that the H.V. Statutory Committee would be given powers by Statutory Instrument following the Act. Obviously this puts us in a very vulnerable position."

25 October 1977 Letter from Director to Secretary Working Group 1 of the Co-ordinating Committee.

"May I suggest a more searching enquiry is required now to begin to quantify that work that is carried out at the moment by all the bodies concerned with education and training. When this has been done, this material would allow a realistic study to be made of the ways in which these activities could, or could not, be carried by the proposed new structure. I have set out my thoughts on one way of collecting this data but there may well be others. As time is short I have taken the liberty of sending a copy to the Chairman of W.G.I. by the same post."

Minutes of meeting Working Group 1, October 1977 - "The majority of the working group were not in favour of a study."

[Note - the question was raised again at the meeting of the Co-ordinating Committee 7 November and 6 December 1977.]

4 November 1977 Delegation from Council led by the Chairman to meet Mr. Moyle, Minister of State. Council's notes of meeting as forwarded to DHSS. Mr. Moyle said:-

"The whole purpose of establishing a Statutory Health Visitor Committee was to retain the present pattern of health visitor education and training. The object of the exercise was to transfer the CETHV into the new machinery and he would say this in Parliament when he introduced the Act. Furthermore, the object of having a Statutory Committee was to preserve some independence of action by discrete bodies. It was very important more Health visitors and District Nurses were produced."

January 1978 Minutes of Council Meeting.

"Members endorsed the Director's concern that the function of the Statutory Committee was not to be clearly spelt out in the Bill the point was made that the Council should not support legislation at any price. Attention was drawn to the fact that preventive services had suffered a great deal from Re-organisation" (of the NHS) "and further erosion in that field must be prevented. The Council asked that firm assurances should be obtained regarding the powers to be given to the Statutory Committee which should not be less than those vested in the Council."

22 February 1978 Minutes of Council Meeting. Reference - Study of the "Position Paper" supplied by the Health Departments - the following Resolution was passed by Council to be forwarded to the Minister by the Chairman and to be taken to the meeting of the Co-ordinating Committee on 27 February.

"The Council endorses much of the philosophy underlying the intentions of the proposed Bill but is nevertheless of the opinion that the mechanism proposed by the Bill for the Education and Training of Health Visitors is not sufficiently specific. Further time is required to elaborate the principles and practice of unification in general, and, in particular, to decide how education for prevention shall be safeguarded and developed.

The Council while appreciating the efforts of the Government to implement the recommendations of the Briggs Report takes the view that the proposed Bill does not guarantee the achievement of those generally accepted recommendations of the Briggs Report. The Council therefore has reluctantly decided that it cannot support the Bill in the form described in the Position Paper.

"However, the Council is anxious that the considerable progress that has been made throughout the last year should not be lost and asks that immediate steps should be taken to continue discussions aimed towards the achievement of a more coherent and integrated education for the nursing profession."

The motion was carried by 12 votes for, 6 votes against and 1 abstention, 1 member leaving before the vote was taken.

[Note - This Resolution was re-affirmed by Postal Ballot October 1978, showing 20 in favour of the Resolution and 5 in favour of the proposed Legislation as it stood. No answers were received from 5 members and there was 1 abstention]

19 July 1978 Minutes of Council Meeting.

"In April Council had agreed that the Director might discuss with the other Bodies concerned the idea of a Federation as an alternative to the structure at present being discussed. The Director had raised this possibility following the May meeting of Working Group 1. The National Union of Public Employees and the RCN" (representatives) "had reacted strongly against, but the CMB (England and Wales) had said it was willing to discuss the possibility."

12 October 1978 Letter from Chairman to the Minister of State.

"We feel it would be helpful if the Government could publish a White or perhaps a Green Paper setting out the case for change and the Government proposals."

19 October 1978 Minutes of Council Meeting.

This meeting was attended by Mr. R.B. Hodgetts, Under Secretary DHSS at the invitation of the Chairman.

The Director reported:

"The CMB (E & W) had written to the Minister stating their past and present concern over the proposed legislation and offering to support the idea of a Federation as suggested by the CETHV. In the discussions of the Co-ordinating Committee all members who spoke - with the exception of two - reaffirmed their inability to support the Bill in the form they had understood it had currently taken. The CETHV was worried by the fact that the profession clearly knew very little about the proposed legislation."

Council Meeting minutes continued:

"The Director was congratulated on the way in which she had expressed this concern in an article published in the Nursing Times." (12 October 1978) (Ref. 16)

Replying to questions raised concerning the wording of the DHSS paper "The Statutory Framework" (which) clearly stipulated that the statutory HV Committee would exercise delegated powers,

Mr. Hodgetts responded:

"With hind-sight the use of the term delegated powers was unwise. Health Visitors and Midwives could not be excluded from the Bill which would in any event go forward subject to the provision of Parliamentary time. It was not a practical proposition for the Council to ask the Minister to 'opt out'."

Council Meeting minutes continued:

"It was difficult to understand how it could be maintained that the phrase the 'exercise of delegated powers' did not mean what it said."

[1 November 1978 - The Queen's Speech - included the Nurses, Midwives and Health Visitors Bill followed by the 1st Reading on 2 November:]

[Nursing Times October 1978; 'Norma Batley is facing wide-spread criticism over her controversial article describing her doubts about the workability of the proposed Briggs Legislation.']

1 November 1978 Letter from Chairman to Mr. Moyle.

"My Council has asked me to write to you again indicating it had re-endorsed the Resolution which had been passed on 22 February 1978. The very clear majority of members of Council still fear the absence of delegated powers for the proposed Statutory Committee for Health Visitors could at worst make it impossible for the hard-won standards for Health Visitors to be maintained in the future."

1, 2 & 9 November 1978 Chairman to Director by phone:

"I think we should send the Resolution with a short explanatory introduction to MPs soon after the publication of the Bill. Try and get Clause 7 better."

[Clause 7 referred to the proposed Health Visitors Joint Committee - the subject of much debate.]

8 November 1978 Letter from Director to all Council Members.

"Since the 1st Reading, the enclosed letter has been sent to every MP and the enclosed paper 'Points for Concern' produced after a meeting of a small group of Council Members which had before

(Ref 16) Nursing Times 12 October 1978

it comments on the Bill from the Council's solicitor. Efforts are being made to arrange a small deputation to meet the Health Group of the Parliamentary Labour Party and with Dr. Gerard Vaughan (Conservative) using 'Points for Concern'. We are also in touch with the HVA, the CMB (E & W), and the Standing Conference of Health Visitor Training Centres."

Extract from a Letter from Director to members of the Council Working Group on the Briggs Legislation at this time.

"I fear I must report almost complete failure in winning over the meeting at the DHSS yesterday on many of the points you raised. I took the precaution of 'phoning 3 likely sympathisers, letting them know in advance that I was going to raise the notion of a White or a Green Paper. All three agreed the profession knew nothing of what was going on; all three agreed to support the idea of a published paper. At the meeting I took my cue from another speaker who mentioned the profession's ignorance of events and said I had been asked to put forward the idea of a Green or a White Paper so that the profession might be best informed. The Secretariat immediately squashed this idea by saying this would delay legislation and what was the point anyway."

28 November 1978 Press Release DHSS - "Nurses' Bill, Mr. Moyle announces new safeguards for Midwives."

"Mr. Moyle will hold meetings with representatives of the Health Visitors later this week."

28 November 1978 Letter from Director to Council Members.

"You will be interested to know that an amendment to Clause 7" (ref. The Health Visitors Joint Committee) "Has already been tabled by Mr. Pavitt MP (Labour) in line with our thinking and I understand the HVA amendment which is much in the same spirit as our own is to be tabled by Dr. Vaughan (Conservative)"

6 December 1978 Letter from Director to Council Members.

"You will wish to know that the CETHV delegation met Mr. Moyle on 30 November led by Dr. Clifford Butler and on 4 December led by Dr. Oliver White" (Council Member).

"On the first occasion the Minister had no new material to discuss with us and we were told to come back on 4 December 1978. On 4 December it was evident that the Minister had had considerable internal consultation in the meantime and had made up his mind that he was not prepared himself to put forward an amendment to Clause 7."

15 December 1978 Telephone from Director to Chairman following attendance at the House of Commons Committee B, Reference Clause 7.

"It had been generally agreed that this Clause was not satisfactory. There had been high praise for the CETHV. The amendments were not agreed but the matter could be raised again. Mr. Moyle says he is prepared to look at any form of words agreed by the Co-ordinating Committee and suggests the professions get together. The Director intends to start with Informal meeting with Mr. Rye, RCN."

[Later - Mr. Rye invited to Council Offices].

24 January 1979 Minutes of Council Meeting.

"The Nurses, Midwives and Health Visitors Bill had been published on 2 November 1978. The Bill had received an unopposed 2nd Reading in the House of Commons on 13 November, but a number of members on both sides had declared their sympathy with the CETHV point of view and their intention to press in the Committee stage for the Bill to be amended on the lines advocated by the CETHV."

25 January 1979 Letter from Chairman to Minister of State.

"The Council has asked me to write to you conveying its present views and explain the basis of the discussions with the other bodies which we are planning during the next few days. There is talk that to accept our amendment would be to make a 'concession' to a minority group. However, we feel we are making very substantial concessions in our amendment to Clause 7 relative to our present position under existing legislation."

April 1979 Minutes of Council Meeting.

"Mr. Moyle, the Minister, had refused to accept the proposed changes to Clause 8 (formerly Clause 7). He had, however, given an undertaking that if the various groups could reach substantial agreement on a 'better solution' the Government would write it into the Bill during the passage through the House of Lords. Representatives of the Council, the RCN, the HVA and Standing Conference had discussed the situation on the 13 February 1979 and agreed a simpler amendment than that originally proposed by the RCN. The amendment had been discussed at the meeting of the Briggs Co-ordinating Committee on 5 March 1979 but had not been approved. However, an alternative version had been agreed."

[*April 1979* N.M. & H.V. Bill 3rd Reading passed by House of Commons.

May 1979 General Election - change from Labour to Conservative Government.]

17 October 1979 Minutes of Council Meeting.

"In July 1979, Council had been informed that the new Ministers were considering the question of implementing the Act in the light of current financial and manpower resources. Council had before it 2 letters dated 2 August and 17 October 1979 from Dr Vaughan, Minister of State (Health). In the first letter Dr. Vaughan had said that he had decided to defer the establishment of the new Central Council and National Boards to allow time to consult widely on matters such as membership. Dr. Vaughan proposed to review the position in 12 months' time and to decide then in the light of progress made in the economic situation, at what date it would be appropriate to introduce the appropriate subordinate legislation. In the second letter the Minister had stated that the reaction to his first letter had left him in no doubt about the strength of feeling and disappointment about the deferment of a decision of implementation for a year - the Minister decided to arrange for an Order to be laid in Parliament."

[The Council had no opportunity to record its view on the Minister's first letter before the second letter was received on the morning of Council Meeting.]

"In discussion, members expressed regret at the Minister's change of mind, although they were aware he had been under pressure to act soon. Members decided a letter should be sent which would 'ask him to endorse the statement made by the Minister of State (Health) in the previous Government - that he said he was sure that arrangements could be made to ensure that the staff would move over in a body to the Health Visiting Joint Committee' " (it was) "noted with disappointment that there was as yet no mention that additional moneys would be provided to improve the education and training of Nurses, Midwives and Health Visitors"

16 July 1980 Minutes of Council Meeting.

"Members noted the 2 papers - relating to the constitution of the National Boards - with effect from 15 September 1980 and of The Central Council from 1 November 1980. Members were informed that in a letter to the Minister of State (Health) dated 5 June 1980 the Chairman has asked that the Council should be recognised as the 'Shadow' Health Visiting Joint Committee. Dr. Vaughan had replied on 7 June 'he did not consider it would be right'. Members were further informed that the Council's Solicitor had advised that if, during this interim period, any of the new bodies appeared to be about to take some steps relating to Health Visiting without due consultation it would be the duty of the Council to draw the attention of the bodies concerned and of the DHSS to the provision of Section 8 (3) of the Act."

SECTION 5 SUPPLEMENT 2

An Example of the "Record of Events" as included in papers for Council Meeting March 1979

BRIGGS LEGISLATION

CETHV - RECORD OF EVENTS - 9th JANUARY to 12th MARCH 1979

A. *OFFICIAL BUSINESS*

IN PARLIAMENT

7th February	3rd Reading, House of Commons
19th February	Attendance at 2nd Reading, House of Lords
13th March	Attendance at Committee Stage, House of Lords

MATERIAL FORWARDED TO MPs AND MEMBERS OF THE HOUSE OF LORDS

2nd February	Material to Mr. Thorne
5th February	Papers to MPs for Report Stage
14th February	Papers to 200 Members of the House of Lords
	Letters and selected enclosures to Lords approached by Chairman
16th February	Letter of thanks to Lords - material sent to four front benchers
12th March	Letters to Lord Sandys and Baronesses Elliot, Vickers and Young
	Letters to Lords contacted by Chairman
	Letters to other members of the House of Lords

MEETING WITH MPs AND MEMBERS OF THE HOUSE OF LORDS

16th January	Conservative MPs
1st February	Labour MPs (Chairman, RCN representative, NBB and HDT)
	Conservative MPs
15th February	House of Lords - Conservative spokesmen, at invitation of HVA

OTHER MEETINGS

5th March	Co-ordinating Committee

B. *INTERNAL ACTION AT CLIFTON HOUSE*

TELEPHONE CALLS

9th January	District Nurses
10th January	Miss Hall, RCN
11th January	Mrs. Latham (Council Member)
20th January	CMB

	HVA
	Panel of Assessors
	Mrs. Croft (DHSS)
25th January	A University
	DHSS
	RCN
	House of Commons
	Solicitor
26th January	Council Members
	HVA
29th January	MPs
1st February	Mrs. Croft (DHSS)
2nd February	GNC
	HVA
	Miss Gough) Standing Conference - Representatives
	Miss Jack) of Health Visitor Training Centres
5th February	HVA
	Dr. Kratz (Nursing Times)
8th February	House of Lords (for lists)
	HVA- invited to attend meeting at House of Lords and arrangements for pre meeting
12th February	Council Members - reactions to 3rd Reading
	Lord Wolfenden (Former Chairman CTHV)
13th February	Lord Wolfenden
16th February	HVA
	RCN
19th February	HVA
	Nursing Times
20th February	HVA
	Mr. Rye, RCN
	Nursing Times (Amendment and explanation)
22nd February	DHSS (re. agenda for meeting on 5th March)
	HVA
	RCN
27th February	DHSS (Re. wording)
12th March	LordWolfenden
	Lord Hunter of Newington

DISCUSSIONS

17th January	Position discussed with PAO and PPA - Tactics for approach to Lords
18th January	Staff Discussion on policy for Council Meeting
8th February	Discussion with Chairman on strategy for Lords
15th February	Miss Jack on description of HV Course

MEETINGS

24th January	Council Meeting
5th February	CMB
7th February	Regional Nursing Officers - Council's attitude explained
13th February	RCN, HVA, Standing Conference representative on revised amendment
22nd February	Informal meeting with Mr. Rye, RCN

MATERIAL TO COUNCIL MEMBERS

6th March	Letter to Council Members
12th March	Letter to Council Members

OTHER

29th January	Preparation of Statement
2nd February	Preparation of papers for all MPs Communicated with Mr. Rye, RCN, and Mr. Parrott, DHSS
9th February	Preparation of paper for Lords
19th February	Letter with amendment to Miss Friend and Mr. Parrott, DHSS
21st February	Preparation of Chart - likely voting at Co-ordinating Committee
26th February	Preparation of paper for Co-ordinating Committee, and despatch
6th March	Contacted Council's Solicitor
9th March	Statement to Standing Conference (of Health Visitor Training Centres)

SECTION 5 SUPPLEMENT 3

Articles and Papers relating to the Briggs Legislation

CETHV Bulletin

Autumn 1975	"Implementation of Briggs"
Spring 1978	"The Briggs Business"
Winter 1978	"The Bill"
Spring 1979	"From the Visitors' Gallery" "Straight Down the Middle"

Nursing Times

9 March 1978	"Big is beautiful"
12 October 1978	"The Briggs Legislation: Is this what is wanted?"
12 April 1979	"Over to You"
7 June 1979	Contribution to "Tales of Mystery and Suspense, or How the Briggs Bill reached the Statute Book"

Booklets supplied by the Council for the use of MPs

"Points for Concern" 7 November 1978

"For use at the Committee Stage - a sequel to 'Points for Concern'' 23 November 1978

"Papers supplied by the CETHV to members of Standing Committee B" 1 February 1979

Also Papers to members of the House of Lords 14 February 1979

SECTION 5 SUPPLEMENT 4

Quotations from the Press

The Times 13 November 1978

"Training health visitors. *From Dr. C.C. Butler, FRS*

Sir, New structure for nursing profession. Your report of the speech by Mr. Roland Moyle, Minister of State (November 7) on this subject prompts me to respond in my capacity as Chairman of the Council for the Education and Training of Health Visitors, especially as the second reading of the Nurses, Midwives and Health Visitors Bill is due, I understand, on November 13.

Mr. Moyle is, of course, correct in stating that some sections of the profession are not happy with the proposals in the Bill. As far as my Council is concerned, our record has been clear and consistent. While disappointed with the Report of the Committee on Nursing (Briggs 1972), not least because little attention was paid to the new educational opportunities for nurses following the introduction of courses for health visitors in universities and polytechnics, the Council nevertheless offered to cooperate with nursing and midwifery educationalists in some form of federation. At the same time, it asked for an assurance that health visitor education and training would be safeguarded.

The fear that our courses might not now be safeguarded led to the Council adopting a resolution in February 1978 (recently reaffirmed) in which regretfully it was unable to support the Government proposals for legislation. At the same time, my Council offered to work towards a more coherent integration of the educational opportunities for the nursing profession than is the case at present. The Council asked me furthermore to write to Mr. Moyle and now to all MPs drawing their attention to our concern.

While a layman in terms of nursing education, I myself have asked Mr. Moyle on more than one occasion for a White Paper on his radical proposals for all to study but, unfortunately, he was unable to do more than provide a Position Paper for limited circulation. My own first reactions on reading the Bill which was presented to Parliament on November 2 are surprise at finding so little said about the long term educational objectives of the new Central Council and concern that the role of the proposed Health Visiting

Joint Committee is not defined nor is its membership largely drawn from practising health visitors.

With the future of the education of nurses, midwives and health visitors at stake, surely more time should now be given to allow for discussion by the profession before the Bill is debated in Parliament?

Yours sincerely,

CLIFFORD BUTLER, Chairman, Council for the Education and Training of Health Visitors, Euston Road, NW1.

November 9."

[Note - this was the final edition of the "Times" before a prolonged shut-down.]

Nursing Times 16 November 1978

"Opposition Health Spokesman, Dr. Gerard Vaughan, told MPs 'We have said we would welcome a Briggs Bill, provided the Nurses, Midwives and Health Visiting professions are reasonably agreed. They are not agreed.' "

Nursing Times 16 November 1978 Radical Midwives in Protest over Briggs

"The Association of Radical Midwives fears the Briggs Bill if implemented will make midwives subordinate to general nurses, deprive them of independent status, lower midwifery teaching standards and produce inadequately trained midwives."

Nursing Times 22 November 1978 Letter from Chairman of Standing Conference of Health Visitor Training Centres

"I write to you again reiterating the points of concern raised in my letter of the 30th January 1978. Our intention is not only to safeguard the present high educational standards of training for future health visitors, but also to be in a position to work for similar educational opportunities for our colleagues."

Nursing Times 22 November 1978 Reference Second Reading of the Bill

"It was the health visitors who came out best. Their protagonists spoke intelligently and forcefully showing they understood the way health visitors felt about being swallowed up in a vast new structure."

Nursing Times 23 November 1978 "Special Report"

Member for Northampton North:

"Instead of patting itself on the back about the extent of consultation the Department should look why the outcome is looking somewhat disastrous."

Nursing Times 23 November 1978 Letter from Miss J. Coombes, RMN, SRN, RNT

"It is all very disturbing but the most disturbing aspect of all remains the attitude of the senior nurses concerned who seem to demand carte blanche to do whatever they wish and to expect unquestioning acceptance from their colleagues."

Nursing Times 7 December 1978 Health Visitors fail to win new Briggs amendment

"At the start of the Committee stage Dr. Gerard Vaughan, the main Opposition spokesman, said 'The Bill is not the un-controversial Bill we were led to believe it to be'."

Nursing Mirror 14 December 1978 Royal College of Nursing - "Will try to halt the Briggs Bill if ... "

"Senior nurse members of the Royal College of Nursing this week threatened to pull all the stops out to prevent the Briggs Bill becoming law if attempts by minority groups 'to alter the Bill's flexibility' were successful."

Midwives Chronicle and Nursing Notes December 1978

Quoting, "Letter to the Minister from the Chairman, Central Midwives Board, England and Wales."

"My Board would first wish to reiterate misgivings they have expressed both verbally and in writing to the Department of Health since the publication of the Briggs Report in 1972."

Nursing Mirror 18 January 1979 Spotlight on News

"It is a supreme irony that the proposed Briggs Bill which has been the rallying cry for the nursing profession for some time now has thrown nurses into bitter anomosity and disunity. Shortly before Christmas, the RCN bowed to pressure and suggested a compromise on the controversial Clause 7 (later 8). Mrs. Wyndham-Kaye (General Secretary, HVA) commented, 'Personally I think Briggs is a very bad Bill. The atmosphere which was already becoming highly charged was not improved by a letter sent out on December the 4th by the Royal College of Nursing General Secretary, Catherine Hall, urging members to lobby MPs to allow "no further concessions to specialist interests".

The RCN has, however, attempted to heal some of the wounds by proposing its concessions to the health visitors on Clause 7."

Nursing Times 15 February 1979 Leader. "In the lap of the Lords"

"Time is running out. Behind the scenes attempts to amend the health visiting Clause so that health visitor education is protected without undermining the powers of the Central Council have so far failed. The indications are that while the RCN and the two health visiting bodies are not too far from agreement, convincing the GNC's. the midwives and the Unions is another matter. I have found it hard this week to find anyone with much enthusiasm left for the Bill."

Nursing Mirror 15 February 1979

"Attempts to safeguard the interests of health visitors were dropped in the House of Commons after a pledge from the Government to make further efforts to reach agreement. Mr. Moyle said he hoped the issue would be resolved in the Lords.

"Stan Thorne, proposing new Clause 8 (re. Joint Committees), said, 'The old Clause had left health visitor training "at the mercy of" the general training system. It is surely no more than common justice that they should be allowed to ensure the future of their own education and training.' "

Nursing Times 1 March 1979 "News"

"The first thing the Co-ordinating Committee will discuss will be a new amendment to the controversial Clause 8 agreed by the RCN, the HVA, the CETHV and the Standing Conference of Health Visitor Training Centres."

Nursing Mirror 9 March 1979

"Health Visitors have won their vital amendment to the Briggs Bill. The Minister was reported afterwards as saying he was delighted by the bridge-building accomplished by various organisations in overcoming a difficult problem."

SECTION 5 SUPPLEMENT 5

The Author's Analysis of Related Influences and Events

During the passage of the 1979 Act, many influences were brought to bear and many events occurred which are worthy of recording. While the following list is in no way comprehensive, the selection that has been made was seen by the Author as being of particular significance and is based on firsthand experience. As far as possible, the information included is supported by documentary evidence.

The Influence of the Health Departments

The previous Sections have illustrated the fact that insofar as legal powers were granted to a Statutory Body the direct involvement of the Health Departments was limited. Indirectly, of course, the Departments' influence continued in respect, for example, of the control of "cash limits", the "establishment of Staff", and might (or might not) be felt as the result of changes in Government policy. At this time when legislation was under review, however, the staff of the Government Departments were in a very powerful position indeed. In the case of the Briggs Report and the sequels, the Health Departments could, for example, select the members of the Briggs Committee which by the nature of things was liable to influence the outcome; accept or ignore the responses received to documents circulated for comment; arrange the agenda for the meetings (e.g. of the Co-ordinating Committee) and advise the Minister at every stage. Finally, when the Act was passed it was the Interdepartmental Group composed of Civil Servants and Nursing Officers from the Health Departments who were to 'set the wheels' in motion prior to the establishment of the Central Council and National Boards. It was also for the staff of these Government Departments to advise on which part of parts of the Act were to be implemented initially.

Later too, no doubt, the offices of the Health Departments would have some 'say' in the appointment of the Chairmen and of the Chief Officers of the new Central Council and National Boards, which again was likely to have some influence on the ways in which the 1979 Act was implemented. All in all, it would be difficult to find another moment in history when the staff of the Health Departments (Departments geared to supplying Health and Social Services rather than Education) were able to influence the future of Nursing, Midwifery and Health Visiting education and training to such and extent.

One result of the 1979 Act has been to ensure the continuing involvement of the Health Departments, not least because of the dependence on financial provision from that source. Their influence, indeed, might be considerably increased as the new Act includes over 20 references to powers in the hands of the Secretary of State. If disputes arise, therefore, which are referable to the Secretary of State, the Health Departments can, ipso facto, become the decision-making bodies. Their influence might be felt additionally, if the Departments' representatives are given the position of membership of Central Council and National Boards as is the custom in respect of some of the existing Bodies - rather than the less involved position of 'Assessors' which has been found to be satisfactory by the Council and in many other spheres.

All meetings of the Co-ordinating Committee were attended by a total of (about) 12 officials representing the four Health Departments. No representatives attended from the Education Departments.

Changes that had taken place since the Publication of the Briggs Report in 1972

The Co-ordinating Committee first met in 1977, but no attempt was made by the Committee to investigate any changes that might have taken place in the interim or if there were any lessons to be learnt from experiences elsewhere. Clearly, a number of significant movements had transpired in those 5 years; examples of these which might have been considered with advantage were:-

(a) The results of constructive talks that had taken place between the Chief Officers of the existing 'bodies' in London and in Edinburgh, stimulated by the Briggs Report, which were already fostering further mutual understanding. (As some Civil Servants were prepared to admit at a later stage, there was no reason why this co-operation could not have continued to grow without any major changes in legislation.)

(b) The increasing number of courses for Nurses, Midwives and Health Visitors which had become established in Institutes of Higher and Further Education; on the whole arrangements were working well, offering a wider educational opportunity to these students than had been experienced before. (Where difficulties had occurred, it was usually traceable to inadequate communication on the part of the examining body concerned.) Furthermore, the move into 'Education' had given Health Visitors and other the opportunity to prove their ability and become recognised alongside a wide range of professions on equal terms.

(c) The Professions Supplementary to Medicine, for example Radiographers, Chiropodists, and Teachers of Physiotherapy, had taken advantage of the expansion of Higher and Further Education facilities during this period and, as a consequence, were finding new ways of developing their education and training.

(d) The publication of the Briggs Report had coincided with the institution in the policy of the Department of Education and Science to phase out 'Monotechnic' - i.e. educational institutions, such as Teacher Training Colleges where students of one profession had been trained in insolation.

(e) The experience of the Central Council for Education and Training in Social Work in bringing together forms of training for specialised workers. This could have had some relevance to the new proposals for Nurses, Midwives and Health Visitors.

(f) Nurse 'students' were by now the only large group whose training remained outside the Education System.

Problems of Terminology, Size and Attitudes

The Nursing, Midwifery and Health Visiting professions have different antecedents and to some extent separate subsequent histories and have been described in many Health Department publications over the years as distinct occupations. At the same time, their education and training programmes have been very different and practitioners have described themselves in terms of membership of one of the three professions.

Significantly too, they are recognised by the public under these three separate titles. However, all may on occasions describe themselves as qualified nurses. To this extent the use of the umbrella term 'nursing' could be felt to be correct. Some of the problems that arose during the meetings of the Co-ordinating Committee centred round confusion as to whether, the term 'nursing' was used in a collective sense with all in partnership or whether, as appeared to be the case on occasions, this indicated that the nurses per se were taking the prime position as leaders and others were appendages and were expected to fit into plans in a subsidiary position. For professions as well established as Midwifery and Health Visiting, this possibility of dominance by others was clearly unacceptable and the suggestion heard at the DHSS that the Bill should be called 'The Nursing Professions' Bill' was immediately rejected by the Midwives present, closely followed by the Health Visitors, and thereafter the title including all the names of the three professions was accepted without dispute.

In the same way, confusion at times appeared to arise out of the great disparity of numbers involved. While the GNC (E & W) could claim pride of place in terms of numbers of students, it was in no way evident to representatives of other organisations that the opionion of the GNC should necessarily carry most weight. Arguably, nurses (per se) could be - and frequently were - the least prepared in terms of training and of experience of the three professions. Neither did it mean, furthermore, that plans which might be carried out happily on a national basis for the large numbers of 'student' nurses were necessarily the best pattern for smaller numbers (unfortunately labelled as 'minority groups') such as Health Visitors and District Nurses.

In these ways and others there were apparent very different considerations, which if recognised as such, could have been the subject of objective debate. Debate, however, was not encouraged by Health Department representatives who reminded the meetings frequently that the Bill had to meet the Parliamentary Time Table, and business was carried forward on the basis of statements expressing the interests of the individual organisations. To raise questions for further consideration, whether on general or specific matters, was as unpopular as it was unrewarding.

The attitudes displayed during the business of the Co-ordinating Committee and Working Parties were in stark contrast to those experienced when Council representatives met with MPs of both parties. Because of their wide experience Members understood immediately and needed no persuasion at all to be convinced of the difficulties being experienced by a small group within a large structure.

Apparent Handicaps to the Interests of Health Visitors

While the integrity of all those in positions of influence was unquestioned, in practical terms the interests of Health Visitors appear to have been at a disadvantage throughout the Briggs negotiations in a number of ways. These handicaps have included:-

1. There were three Registered Nurse Tutors on the Briggs Committee but there was no Health Visitor Tutor - neither was there a representative from Higher and Further Education conversant with the development of Health Visitor (and other) courses within the Education System.
2. The Briggs Report contained extensive coverage of the work of the General Nursing Councils and the Joint Board of Clinical Nursing Studies, but made only scant reference to the Council's work which had been recognised already as significant by some senior nurses and educationalists.
3. The Council entered into the negotiations which were to lead to the 1979 Act in the expectation that there was to be a Statutory Health Visitors Committee 'with delegated powers'. This provision was later removed - a DHSS representative stating that this phrase was seen "with hindsight to have been unwise".
4. While the Council (and it is understood the CMB for England and Wales) had made clear its disagreement in writing on a number of occasions, the Bill was presented as 'Non-Controversial', MPs of both main parties later expressing suprise as the facts became known to them.
5. After meeting with the representatives of the Midwives, which led to the announcement of 'new safeguards for midwives', the Minister of State arranged "similarly" to meet the representatives of the Health Visitors, but when this occurred he had no suggestions to make or explanation to give.

[Note: If an acceptable offer had been made at this stage, the subsequent representations by the Council and the Health Visiting profession might have been unnecessary,]

6. The only evidence of the work of the existing 'bodies' asked for at any stage by the Co-ordinating Committee (or its Working Parties) was that of those concerned with Nurse training (per se).
7. After the 1979 Act was passed, the Inter-departmental Group of Civil Servants and Nursing from the four Health Departments, who were to prepare the ground for the establishment of the Central Council and National Boards, had no Health Visitor representative.

While these 'handicaps' may have been the results of oversights, or based on the assumption that nurses could express the views of health visitors also, nevertheless they contributed substantially to the growing unease, unease which might have been felt equally, for example, if those responsible for nurse training had found themselves similarly overlooked.

And lastly there was the psychological handicap of knowing that, in spite of the interest shown in some quarters, in practice none of the Chief Nursing Officers nor the influential spokesman for the RCN was a qualified Health Visitor and - in contrast to the close involvement some had had as members, of the GNC (England & Wales) and the JCBNS, for example - none had had firsthand experience of the meetings of the CETHV.

The Influence of Professional Organisations and Trades Unions

It will be appreciated that it was the Royal College of Nursing that asked that the "enquiry into nursing" should take place, that welcomed the Report in enthusiastic terms and continued over the years to signify in its publications that this new Act would be 'a good thing'. And undoubtedly a professional organization of this size and standing had a substantial influence in many quarters, including the Government Departments. It was apparent from the reports of the meetings of the Co-ordinating Committee that the RCN conceded with great reluctance to the idea of any Statutory Committees within the provisions of the 1979 Act. It was influenced ultimately, however, by the action group of District Nurses among its membership and, at a very late stage, when the passage of the Act itself was in doubt, by a sharp reminder of the need to represent the interests of its Health Visitor members too. This reaction by HV members to a controversial letter distributed by the General Secretary of the RCN in which reference was made to 'concessions' to specialist groups, may be seen by historians in future as having provided a 'watershed', for the meeting that followed between representatives of the RCN, HVA and the Council resulted in an agreed amendment which led on to a modified version accepted by all members of the Co-ordinating Committee. These events might be interpreted by some as the Royal College of Nursing rescuing the Act when a breakdown seemed distinctly possible or it might be seen by others as a belated effort on the part of the Royal College to consider the wishes of not only its Nurse members but also of District Nurses and Health Visitors. The facts, however, show that without doubt the Royal College of Nursing with its historic links with the GNC and the JBCNS, had a leading role before, during and after the passing of the 1979 Act.

With the business of the meetings of the Co-ordinating Committee centred on the structure of the proposed new Statutory Organisations and not on educational issues the input from the Professional Organisations and from the Trades Unions was substantial - not least because the Minister of State who Chaired the first meeting, Mr. Roland Moyle, was himself sponsored by a Trades Union as an MP. In practice, two Unions spoke up for the interests of the Psychiatric Nurses, the Royal College of Midwives for the Midwives (not necessarily with the same views as the CMB), and the HVA for the Health Visitors. The CETHV had good reason to be grateful to the independent but totally supportive action taken by the HVA during these times. Other organisations which 'spoke up' for HV education and training included the Standing Conference of Health Visitor Training Centres, which organised planned campaigns, and the Committee of Directors of Polytechnics. All these efforts, as well as those of countless individual HVs, resulted in a notable and consistant 'lobbying' of MPs, and the impression made included in the Hansard records of the readings of the NMHV Bill.

It may be seen as significant that some District Nurses and some Midwives in particular also formed pressure groups and mounted a an effective lobbying of MPs when it became clear their wishes were not being met. Indeed, all these groups and others 'lobbied.' MPs during the passage of the Bill, which in itself was indicative of the lack of satisfaction with the work of the Co-ordinating Committee and the subsequent provisions in the Bill.

The Position of the Chief Officers of the Statutory and Non-Statutory Bodies

During the time of the meetings of the Co-ordinating Committee, three out of the eight Chief Officers of the statutory and non-statutory bodies retired and it was never possible, in the opinion of the Author, to regain the co-operative relationships enjoyed in 1975. The newcomers joined in the negotiations when all the exisiting organizations were in a poisition of uncertainty and stress and, in any case, as Chief Officers they were bound to present the case for the divergent interests of their own organization. At various times, at their own meetings, however, Chief Officers expressed considerable doubts about the proposed new structure, as was shown in their reaction to the 'Position Paper' circulated by the DHSS to members of the Co-ordinating Committee before the Bill was laid before Parliament.

Notes of the meeting of the London-based Chief Officers on 10 February 1978 stated "the plans for the Bill as revealed in the recent 'Position Paper' were of grave concern to all of us. As Chief Officers

we would do better to speak collectively preferably to being party to an arrangement which all of us knew to be undesirable. It was necessary for us to be constructive and suggest a way forward. The first essential was to consult others'' (i.e. Chief Officers) ''on 20 February and if agreed, it would be necessary to seek a meeting with the Chief Nursing Officer (DHSS) before the Co-ordinating Committee meeting on 27 February.'' At the meeting of all the Chief Officers it was agreed ''none of the options'' (in the 'Position Paper') ''would produce a non-controversial Bill. It was finally agreed that no approach could be made to the Minister; although all members opposed the present 'Position Paper' they did so for varied reasons.''
[The official comments from these organizations and others to the 'Position Paper' were subsequently reported at the meeting of the Co-ordinating Committee.]

The Unanswered Questions

During the meetings of the Co-ordinating Committee and the Working Parties, some major questions were left unanswered and usually when differences of opinion emerged it was stated that ''it would be left for the Central Council and National Boards to decide''.

Examples of these questions were:-
1. What was to be the relative position of the Central Council and National Boards? This question was of particular concern to those with national interests.
2. Who would pay any fees that might be required, the employee or the employer? The two Royal College representatives favoured the former and some Union representatives the latter.
3. Was the plan suggested 'feasible' in terms of work load? This question became the particular concern of the Author who raised the question several times - in particular at Working Group 1.

As evidence had been taken from some, but not all, the existing statutory and non-statutory 'bodies', clearly plans for legislation went forward without regard to the total of ongoing commitments alone which the new structure would have to carry; for example, at no time was the CETHV asked for evidence of the work it was undertaking. The paper offered by the Author suggested, therefore, that basic factual material should be collected from *all* sources. The item was given a late position on the Agenda, introduced without any indication of importance and set aside by the meeting as unnecessary. The Bill went forward, therefore, without any calculation on 'feasibility' other than a theoretical paper produced by the Secretariat when the Chairman of the Committee had mentioned the subject at an early stage which was unsupported by any factual evidence. In other words, it was not known whether the plans were workable having regard to the fact that the Central Council and the National Board members would be in full-time employment.

But, perhaps the most important question of all, was never asked - what was the real purpose of the Act?

An Alternative Plan for a Federation

Mention of the word 'Federation' was recorded first in the Council's comments on the Briggs Report. Later the possibility was 'aired' informally with a group of London-based Chief Officers where it was studied with considerable interest and some enthusiasm and it was agreed that it should be taken to the meeting of all the Chief Officers. At the meeting that followed, however, it was decided not to continue a study of this idea as it would delay legislation.

The plan as far as the thinking had gone, was to retain the existing organisations, updating legislation where required and establishing a Central Council first on a voluntary basis with a view to legislation at a later date. The Central Council would take up the subjects of co-ordinating International affairs, Research, Discipline, Records and Education and other matters of common interest. The object would be to encourage the existing bodies to move further towards overall co-ordination in agreement and at their own pace without fear that particular interests would be overriden. Later, after the Council had asked the Director to put the idea forward, the Chairman informing the Minister and the Director the Chief Nursing Officers, a chance was given for the proposal to be discussed with those who could spare the time to remain after a meeting of the Working Group 1 on 16 May 1978. Again, it was made clear by those who wished to see a new Bill before Parliament within the time-table suggested by the DHSS, that study of another plan would delay legislation and no further action was called for. Finally, the idea was raised again by the Director at a meeting of the Co-ordinating Committee but was dismissed immediately by the Royal College of Nursing representative on the same grounds and was not discussed further.

It is noteworthy, however, that the idea of a Federation received the official support of the CMB (England & Wales) in the autumn of 1978. Additionally, this alternative was commended informally during the passage of the Bill and has continued to be applauded since by a number of individuals at a very high level. History will not now relate whether this alternative plan would or would not have gained ground if presented earlier. But in view of the fact that it appeared originally that a Bill was to go forward incorporating a Health Visitor

Statutory Committee with delegated powers, it had not appeared necessary to suggest the Federation plan in the initial stages.

The Cost in Losses and Gains

If it were possible to add up the total financial costs incurred in the long sequence of events starting with the meetings of the Briggs Committee and continuing up to the time of the establishment of the Central Council and National Boards, the total undoubtedly would be very formidable indeed. Some figures could be found, no doubt, in the files of the Health Department, such as the costs of the meetings of the Co-ordinating Committee, but the exercises (and therefore expenditure incurred) that were generated by such radical proposals among the 'interested parties' would be impossible to trace, spanning as they did nearly ten years in all. As well as the large sums of public monies involved, it is known that professional organisations, unions, and individuals, from the time of preparing evidence to the Briggs Committee in 1970 onwards, went to considerable lengths to make their views known and all this cost money.

Another cost, which again would be impossbile to trace, would be in terms of 'man hours'. Alongside Department meetings were an unspecified number of official and informal meetings ranging from those of (say) working groups of Council members to special meetings of the various professions involved and individual meetings with MPs by delegates or by concerned individuals. As a consequence of this, there was a second incalculable cost as tasks were left undone in order to give time to these new demands. These costs will continue, no doubt, while the 1979 Act is being implemented.

Another less tangible but important loss must be added; the 'Good Will' experienced among those considering the business in 1975 which was 'lost along the line', as the smaller groups felt themselves threatened.

The gains and losses overall can only be estimated in the years to be. From the reading of the Act, however, it could be suggested that it would be the Health Departments, National interests and the interests of the nursing profession per se who were the first gainers in terms of 'power'. The Act, however, stated the principal function of the Central Council shall be to establish and *improve* standards of training and professional conduct for Nurses, Midwives and Health Visitors and only time will show to what extent this threefold purpose is realised.

When the Act was passed the Council, among many others, immediately offered co-operation and it was universally accepted that ways must now be found to make the new Act work.

SUMMARY

SECTION 1 - MIDDLE YEARS - (Page 1)

External developments (Page 1) had much influence on the work of the Council. Publications by the Health Department and from other sources stressing the importance of 'prevention' and the need for Health Visitors, together with developments in Higher and Further Education were encouraging. At the same time, however, the Reorganisation of the NHS in 1974 which removed the management structure for Health Visitors and the 'pooling' system for Health Visitor students; the Halsbury Report which led to the removal of the financial 'lead' for Field Work Teachers, and the EEC Directives on Midwifery caused substantial threats to Health Visitor education and training. Recruitment to HV courses was immediately affected and has never recovered. Accommodating the larger groups acted in these cases directly to the detriment of the smaller and situations were only retrieved where possible at great costs. The Council had 'taken the tide' establishing courses in Higher and Further Education and relationships with the Institutions continued to develop on the basis of the recognition of responsibilities and mutual respect. The 'Devolution Debate' had stimulated an agreed statement from all four countries that Health Visitor education and training should continue on a U.K. basis. The link between the Government Departments and the Council was maintained satisfactorily by 'Assessors'.

The influence of related professions (Page 7) could be studied in terms of Nurses, of Midwives, or of Health Visitors, taking into account variations in different countries and different points in time. For example, the growth of Social Work had affected the Health Visitors in the early 1970s and now consideration was to be given to the new developments in District Nursing. A joint statement was prepared by the Panel of Assessors for District Nurse Training and the Council for the consideration of the educational institution arranging the two courses. The importance of attitude formation at the student stage was studied further by the Symposium in Nottingham in 1979 arranged in equal partnership between the four bodies responsible for the preparation of General Practitioners, Social Workers, District Nurses and Health Visitors. This exemplified the two-directional pull experienced in the work of the Council; the necessity to consider primary care workers as a whole on the one hand and Nurses engaged in curative services on the other.

The relationship between 'education' and 'service' personnel required continuing attention. There was a further clarification of legal responsibilities between the Council and the educational institutions and Service Managers were involved in the official 'Visitations' to the educational institutions. While it was recognised that variations in local services existed, the Council's policy was to retain the Health Visitor Course as 'basic' and 'general'. Traditionally, Nurse Administrators were involved in the planning of nurse training. The case for the educationalists to contribute to the thinking of the service was a more recent growth. But it was evident that each party could 'spark off ideas' in the other. In the rare cases of complaint that a course had not prepared the Health Visitor for the job, the question should be asked, was it the course or the working situation at fault?

Internal developments. (Page 13)

In 1976 Dr. Clifford Butler, Vice-Chancellor of Loughborough University of Technology, took over the chairmanship of the Council from Professor (now Sir John) Butterfield. The Sixth Council took office in October 1977. While the appointment rather than election of members may seem an anachronism today, the width of experience brought to bear on the Council's business proved invaluable and the mixed membership ensured the element of questioning. Health Visitors themselves comprised about one-third of the membership and some were known to make up to 25-30 attendances a year. The separation from the CCETSW, the appointment of the second Director, and new administrative staff in 1975, provided the moment for new structuring of staff. The problem of different salary scales, accounted for the post of the Principal Professional Adviser being filled only intermittently.

The relationship between Council members and Council staff had some of the features noted between MPs and Civil Servants. In this case care had to be taken to ensure that power always remained in the hands of the members of the Council.

Domestic issues included the consideration of the structure and functions of the staff; the slight modification of former arrangements for centralisation by the establishment of a new office in Edinburgh; the establishment of a Joint Staff Consultative Committee; new conditions of service (later approved by the DHSS) and quarterly meetings of all staff members. The report of an external investigation of salary scales aimed at resolving salary problems, was not accepted by Council. Acute problems of accommodation were resolved in 1977 when the Council moved to new offices within Clifton House offering good working conditions, an appropriate 'image' to visitors and extended opportunities.

SECTION 2 - THE EXERCISE OF POWERS (Page 23)

The Council continued to operate under the terms of the 1962 Act updated now by the addition of two further Statutory Instruments. In practical terms, the Act had provided an exceptionally wide range of responsibilities spanning recruitment, pre-requisite qualifications, the provision and approval of Health Visitor Courses, further education and research. From the experience of the Council it was clear that it was the exceptional range of responsibilities along with related developments that generated the volume of work. Apart from the mounting concern over the ommission of disciplinary powers, there was no evidence to suggest the Council itself would have wished to instigate any major changes in legislation. A Working Party was set up to investigate the subject of discipline and its first papers were circulated to the Professional Organisations for comments. The ommission of mention of National Advisory Committees for England and Wales respectively in the 1962 Act was remedied by the establishment of two committees of Council. The meaning of the Act was put to the test in one case when the question of the Council planning courses for School Nurses was referred to the Health Departments for decision. In general, the history of the Council reflects the implementation of a well-worded Act, the interpretation necessarily resting in the hands of Council members and Council staff. Records now showed a substantial volume of action in relation to all the Council's powers, some of which had been noted by others to be of an innovatory or pioneering nature.

The work of the Council Committees and Working Parties - (Page 25)

The methods of working continued in line with the plan described in 'The History of the Council for the Education and Training of Health Visitors' by Elaine Wilkie. Council meetings were held four times a year with 'Extraordinary' meetings additionally on such subjects as the Court Report. The pattern of holding one meeting every second year either in Scotland, Wales or Northern Ireland was continued when possible. The agenda of Council meetings included major policy matters and the reports of the National Advisory Committees and main committees of Council. In 1976 a group was formed of the Chairmen of all the main committees, later to be known as the Chairman's Committee, which had as its terms of reference the duty to formulate and submit to the Council a cohesive policy regarding both external and internal developments in the Council's work both for the short and the long term. The number of co-opted members to Committees never exceeded one-third of the membership and in this way Council members remained in control of all Council's business. Other activities included the formation of a Professional

Organisations Consultative Committee which was composed of representatives of related professional organisations based in England and in Scotland; 'Open Days' for Service Managers; and the Director's informal meetings with Health Visitor Tutors in five centres in the U.K. twice a year, for it was the quality of work 'at the coal face' that was the deciding factor in the success or failure of the conversion of the Council's policies into practice.

On-going commitments, areas of development and matters arising out of external changes - (Page 30)

The work of the Council could be considered in these three inter-related catagories. Matters arising out of external changes could hardly have been more fundamental during this period, the effects of the Re-organisation of the National Health Service, the EEC Directives and the birth of the Nurses, Midwives and Health Visitors Act 1979.

The Strategy Plan and Sequels - (Page 30)

The final separation of this Council from the Central Council for Education and Training in Social Work (November 1974) and the introduction of new staff (Spring 1975) provided a suitable moment for a review of work accomplished so far and a consideration of work still to be done. The 'Strategy Plan' worked out first of all for the benefit of the staff themselves was later taken up in various papers to the Chairman's Committee and to Council. By July 1980, it was reported to Council that all the principal items listed in 1975 had received attention (See Section 2, Supplement 1).

The story of the Council is one of continuing change. The pace of change, due to exceptional circumstances including the uncertainties of the future, was felt at times to place undue pressure on Council Members and Staff as well as Health Visitor Tutors.

Comments from Council - (Page 31)

The 'Middle Years' produced a 'bumper crop' of reports which had relevance to the work of the Council and providing 'Comments' proved to be a very substantial commitment. A new formula was agreed by Council for dealing with these 'Comments' ranging from a letter from the Director to Working Parties of Council Members producing material, first on a national basis and then collectively in Council. When necessary, this involved a half-day or even an 'Extraordinary' meeting of Council before an agreed document was completed. The ultimate effect of these 'Comments' cannot be estimated but strongly expressed views on issues pertinent to HV education and training and its future appear to have been passed over. It is known, however, that favourable observations were made elsewhere regarding 'Council's Comments' on plans for the NHS. The policies revealed in 'Council's Comments' suggest that a comparative study of these alongside those of other professions would reveal ways in which a variety of professions think alike and where they differ.

The Extending Responsibilities - (Page 33)

The Council's work became extended as the widespread 'functions' prescribed under the 1962 Act were further developed in the four countries of the U.K. Additionally the Council was much involved in what proved to be the extensive exercise generated by the preparation for the 1979 Act. In these negotiations Council consistently pursued the twofold policy of offering co-operation with Nurses and Midwives at the same time asking that the education and training of Health Visitors should be safeguarded.

SECTION 3 - MAJOR DEVELOPMENTS - (Page 37)

Even minor changes in connection with the routine work of the Council required time and effort. Stimuli for major development appeared from a number of sources: as a natural sequel to established practice and from the 'Strategy' exercise; from the Health Visitor Tutors; from the requirement for more substantial factual evidence; from School Nurses, as well as from employers. Additionally, the Council was required to respond to proposals arising within the educational institutions themselves.

Further Education - (Page 38)

A comprehensive plan for continuing education for health visitors was the subject of two Council reports in 1977 and 1979. The first included a flowchart which suggested Futher Education and Training in terms of vertical and lateral growth (See Section 3, Supplement 1), included aims and objectives and indicated the importance of progressive staff development linked with performance review. It suggested the basic course should be followed by a variety of ongoing special skills courses and indicated the need for national and local policies. The second concluded with the suggestion for two categories of Further Education Courses and the establishment of a Further Education Liaison Group with representatives from 'Education' and 'Service'.

Health Visitor Tutors' Courses - (Page 39)

The pattern that emerged provided for two major centres and other smaller facilities to meet local needs. Policy decisions were related to the problem of small numbers and to the Council's educational philosophy. Longstanding financial difficulties were studied by the Briggs Co-ordinating Committee which finally recommended that there should be central funding for health visitor tutor students and the involvement of the Council in these arrangements.

Fieldwork Teachers' Courses - (Page 41)

The Council re-designed further the fieldwork teacher courses. Some administrative problems were encountered initially but early reactions to the course itself were favourable. The inhibiting problem of fieldwork teachers' salaries, however, persisted.

Assessors of Supervised Practice Courses - (Page 42)

Local initiative had been taken in some places to provide courses in preparation for this role. The recommendations of the Council's Working Party resulted in a Council provision for courses totalling five days' duration.

Courses in School Nursing - (Page 42)

The possibility of developing a course for School Nurses was first mentioned in Council in 1975. After correspondence with the DHSS, the Council was able in 1977 to offer guidelines to a syllabus for a course in School Nursing and later acted upon the official encouragement given and designed a further course for Nurses caring for the Physically Handicapped Child. By the end of 1980, a number of courses in School Nursing had been approved.

Curriculum Development - (Page 43)

In January 1978 a working party of Education Committee (later expanded to include other representation) was set up to advise on the subject of curriculum development and the early work included the production of a plan of progression, the collection of evidence on job description and the study of behavioural objectives. Alongside this, was the investigation into principals and practice carried out mainly by a group of Health Visitor Tutors with the support of Council's staff, working within the terms of reference prescribed by Education Committee. As it was necessary for a study in detail of the role of the Health Visitor to be undertaken before the study of curriculum development as such could begin, this complex exercise was unlikely to be completed for some time.

Health Visitor Manpower Investigation - (Page 44)

This investigation was initiated by Research Committee in order to find out with greater precision than before the requirements for Student Health Visitor places. The first returns were incomplete but provided some indication of trends which if continued will provide a 'tool' to decision-making never before available.

Other Developments - (Page 45)

Current practices in Institutes of Higher and Further Education were influential in the development of 'Satellite' courses and for the 'Visitations' in connection with the approval of courses. The growth in the variety of courses for which Council's approval was required raised the question of a different form of approval procedure.

Developments undertaken depended on a number of factors not least a touch of imaginative thinking without which none of these advances would ever have taken place.

SECTION 4 - THE ROLE OF A U.K. STATUTORY BODY- (Page 48)

Before any worthwhile account could be given of the role of the Council as a U.K. Statutory Body, it was necessary to appreciate the history of the establishment of the four National Advisory Committees, their individual features and the ways in which they relate to the Council itself.

The 1962 Act had resulted in the establishment of the only Statutory Body to date in this field of work with a range of responsibilities throughout the United Kingdom. Success appeared to be founded on the recognition of two potentially opposing factors, the very real differences between the four countries and the recognition of what was the same in the terms of the Council's business. Differences included cultural patterns, geographical features, legal provision, and the important difference in size. There was considerable variation too in the degree of interest shown in the development of Health Visiting in different localities within each country. Particular features of this U.K. organisation have been summarised under the following headings: Council meetings, membership of committees, communications, National Advisory Committees, individual arrangement, publications, and staffing. The workload of a statutory body which is required to carry out functions on a U.K. basis is considerably greater than that required for a similar assignment on a national basis only. This needs to be reflected in the number of members as well as the numbers of staff.

International Affairs - (Page 52)

Links have revealed a widespread interest in prevention and community care in both advanced and developing countries. If Health Visitors have reason to feel they are 'prophets without honour in their own country', the Council was left in no doubt of the interest overseas. On the evidence of this international interest, the Council proposed in 1979 that consideration should be given to the possibility of an International Conference at an early date.

Public Relations - (Page 53)

The Council has been mindful of the importance of public relations and the third film 'One Step Ahead' was produced in 1979. As well as personal contracts, publications including the 'Bulletin' twice a year and three additional books have been produced (see Section 4, Supplement 1). An unexpected boost arose out of the passage of the 1979 Act when papers for MPs and the responsible lobbying by Health

Visitors themselves left Parliment in little doubt about the activities of the Council and the concern that this kind of provision for education and training should continue.

SECTION 5 - THE PASSAGE OF THE ACT - (Page 55)

A complete history of the passage of the 1979 Act could be compiled only after reference to the records of all those involved. Council papers alone extend from 'Evidence to the Briggs Committee' onwards including, for example, correspondence with the Minister of State (Health), notes of internal and external meetings and contributions to the press.

Unlike some others, Council had expressed disappointment in the Briggs Report, but had from that time onwards consistently stated and pursued the two fold policy of offering co-operation with nurses and midwives and, at the same time, requiring to be assured that the future education and training of Health Visitors would be safeguarded. *'Extracts from Council Papers'* (Section 5 Supplement 1) - (Page 60) include quotations from Council Minutes and Correspondence from the Spring of 1975, when the former Director was able to report at her last attendance that at a meeting with the Government Departments on 26 February "the proposal that the Statutory Committee" "Health Visiting would be a Central Body with continuing responsibility for the U.K. was especially welcome". This was followed later by 'Comments from the Council' on the Health Departments' subsequent publication 'The Statutory Framework' which stated "the Health Visitor Committee should exercise delegated powers in relation to the functions of the Central Council" which was agreed, but the Council registered "grave concern at the very significant change of authority oulined in the new document in relation to the National Boards". At a later stage still, in response to the Departments' first paper to the Co-ordinating Committee, Council commented "the study of the function of the Central Council and National Boards without a concurrent study of the Statutory Committees was unrealistic" and "at a time when the Government is calling for the expansion of the Health Visiting Service, any such move could be catastrophic".

The Director's letter to the Chairman in September 1977 stated, "I have become very disturbed at the trend of events". However, the Council's notes of a meeting with the Minister of State on 4 November 1977 included the following quotation from the Minister: "The whole purpose of the establishment of the Statutory Health Visitors Committee was to retain the present pattern of Health Visitor education and training".

Later quotations included the concern of the Council that the functions of the Council were not to be clearly spelt out in the Bill and the Council's subsequent Resolution, following the study of the Health Departments' Position Paper stated: "The Council therefore has reluctantly decided it cannot support the Bill in the form described". The Director was instructed to discuss with other Bodies the idea of a Federation (later officially supported by the CMB), the Chairman sent a letter to the Minister asking for him to consider issuing a White (or Green) Paper. In October 1978, Mr. Hodgetts, Under-Secretary (DHSS) was invited to attend Council Meeting. In response to questioning he stated with reference to the wording of the Government Paper "The Statutory Framework" that "with hindsight the term 'delegated powers' was unwise". He also indicated that it would not be possible now for the Council to 'opt out' of the new legislation if it so wished.

After the publication of the Bill, there were meetings with MPs of both parties who gave very sympathetic reception to the Council's expressions of concern and offered to table amendments. Also the Department's Press Release of 28 November 1978, announced "new safeguards for midwives" to be followed by a similar meeting with the representatives of Health Visitors. In the event, however, the Minister made no new offers to the Council's delegation.

Later, when the Minister had asked all of those represented on the Co-ordinating Committee to seek a solution, the Council's Chairman wrote to the Minister in January 1979 'explaining the basis of the discussions with other bodies which we are planning in the next few days' and added "we feel we are making very substantial concessions in our amendment to Clause 7 (ref Health Visiting Joint Committee) "relative to our present position under existing legislation". The Minutes of Council Meeting April 1979 stated "an agreement was reached between the HVA, the RCN, the Standing Conference of Health Visitor Training Centres" (and the Council's representatives) "on an amendment which when modified further was accepted by all parties".

Following the General Election in 1979, the incoming Conservative Minister of State (Health) sent two letters - the first indicating his decision to delay the implementation of the 1979 Act and the second stating that as the result of the response he had received, he had decided to arrange for "an order in Parliament". As the second letter was received also before Council Meeting, the CETHV did not record its views on the first. Minutes of Council Meeting on 17 October 1979 however, included "regret at the decision" and asked that a letter be sent asking the Minister to endorse the previous Minister of State's

assurance that "he was sure arrangements could be made to ensure that the staff would move over as a body to the Health Visitors' Joint Committee" and "it was noted with disappointment that there was as yet no mention that additional monies would be provided to improve the education and training of Nurses, Midwives and Health Visitors". A request was made that the Council should be recognised as the "shadow" Health Visiting Joint Committee but this was not granted. Supplements are added under the following headings:-
1. "Extracts from Council Papers" (Page 60); 2. an example of a "Record of Events"; 3. a list of "Articles and Papers relating to the Briggs Legislation"; 4. "Quotations from the Press" and 5. The Author's analysis of "Related Influences and Events" which includes the subjects of "The Influence of the Health Departments", "Changes that had taken place since the publication of the Briggs Report in 1972", "Problems of Terminology", "Apparent handicaps to the interest of Health Visitors", "The Influence of the Professional Organisations and Trades Unions", "The Position of the Chief Officers", "The Unanswered Question", "An Alternative Plan for a Federation" and "The Cost in Losses and Gains".

This account of the "History of the CETHV, Book 2, The Middle Years" is followed by; "Postscript by the Author"

Appendix i Members of Council 1974-1977
ii Members of Council 1977-1980
iii Council
iv Student Numbers

POSTSCRIPT BY AUTHOR

"The past is inspiring, the future is challenging, the present is our responsibility. Let us, therefore, while shouldering these responsible duties, and in the consciousness of the achievements of the past which we have inherited, so plan for the future with wisdom, foresight and integrity, that when succeeding generations look back on us as we ourselves survey the past, then our page of history shall seem no less inspiring than those that have gone before."

Daisy Bridges, ICN Stockholm 1949.

When "Succeeding generations look back", first of all what will they make of the work of the CETHV from 1975 to 1980? Surely they will count among the failures the continuing complaint that the HV courses were overcrowded, that a few centres were still having difficulties in getting the most suitable accommodation and other resources and, of course, the poor record of recruitment. No doubt too, they will note that the HV Certificate, although named as "advanced" in the terminology of the public sector of education, had not yet been linked universally with one of the recognised standards - 'Certificate', 'Diploma' or 'Degree' - neither had the idea of establishing a Chair in Health Visiting even reached the 'drawing-board'.

Perhaps, however, the CETHV which in total will have had a life-span of 20 years only will be credited with some successes. It had established courses for a statutory qualification on a U K basis; it had designed a complete plan for courses of further education; it had taken a lead in encouraging inter-professional understanding between the professions engaged in Primary Care; it had involved those responsible for teaching student HVs in the business of the Council, and it had attempted a manpower planning exercise on a UK basis. But most importantly, the students emerging form the HV courses were in general mature, articulate and skilled practitioners - the result, in the opinion of the HVs themselves of the wider form of education offered in the Universities, Polytechnics and Colleges which the Council had initiated.

But surely too, "those who come after" will recognise the vulnerability of the work of the Council. Comprehensive decisions for Nurses, Midwives and Health Visitors had been made without, it appeared, any built-in protection for smaller groups. Would the removal of a management structure for Health Visitors, which had been one result of the Reorganisation of the National Health Service in 1974, allow for the further development of expertise and "push the frontiers of Health Visiting forward", and could a profession flourish which might offer now no promotion opportunities in Health Visiting per se beyond that of Nursing Officer? Would the loss of a financial lead for the Fieldwork Teacher mean the eventual demise of this worker and the inevitable loss of skill in the practical training of students that would result? Would the fact that the EEC Directives had been implemented without any money being made available to meet the inevitable costs start a downward spiral in recruitment that could not be reversed? What future was there when Service Managers were left with the dilemma of finding moneys for education and for the service from the same fund? All in all, how serious were the Government and the Health Departments about the development of Primary Care or was this to be another case of the U.K. "first in the field", with its long experience of Health Visiting and District Nursing, now being left behind?

And when "succeeding generations look back", what rating will they give the Briggs Report, the preparation for and the eventual provisions of the 1979 Act, and the actions of those who were involved?

Will they begin with the basic question "What was the case for this Act?" If so, no doubt they will see that some, but not all, of the existing Statutory Bodies had been asking for changes in "Their" legislation for some time, also that there were other Non-Statutory Bodies which should now be controlled too by legislation. Added to this, it would be much easier for Health Departments and the administrators of the service, it might seem, to have one comprehensive organisation to deal with. Perhaps too there could have been some individuals or organisations which might - for worthy or less worthy motives - see these changes as a chance to add strength to their particular interests. What may be unclear, however, were the new objectives in terms of education and training which warranted such radical changes in legislation. For a start, they will dismiss as false the persistent impression of the day in some quarters that this legislation was necessary in order that there should be co-ordination of planning between those responsible for the various branches of education and training. They will know that there had been already many examples of joint thinking between a variety of Statutory Bodies over the years in the Integrated, Degree and Diploma course developments, and that the Briggs Report itself had had a marked effect in stimulating this thinking further in some places without any changes in the law. They will see too the problems faced by educators who had to consider such variables as applied studies, the depth of knowledge required and the time available for the course. There was more to the business of linking courses than simply "knocking heads together''. Clearly too there was no reason why collective thinking could not have continued, neither was there any bar to the preparation of a comprehensive register of qualified staff, if needed, by co-operation between the established organisations. It will be understood, however, that some up-dating would have been required in any case and, perhaps, for administrators in particular this seemed a good moment to tidy things up. Futhermore, human nature appears to dictate that people are keener ''to build a new Town Hall than to repair the highways''. But whether or not there was ever a worthwhile educational argument for such radical change can only be judged at a later date. Only the future, however, will show whether a tidy administrative structure is compatible with the diversity of pioneering ventures so essential to progress in education. The questions might be asked even now (hypothetically at least): Would the initiatives taken by the CETHV have occurred within the framework of a 1979 type Act? And what new educational opportunities will the 1979 Act offer which were unavailable before?

No doubt, too, our successors will ask ''What were the root causes of the disputes that arose during the passage of the Bill?'' and ''How was it that an exercise that started in a spirit of co-operation ended up for settlement in the House of Lords?'' Certainly, it will be seen that all of those involved had their own particular hopes and fears. For example, the relationship between the Central Council and the National Boards was the cause of concern to those who wished to retain as much power as possible on a national basis. (It was sympomatic of this fear that at one stage the Secretariat placed the National Boards above the Central Council on the paper prepared for the Co-ordinating Committee.) They would see, too, that the comments on documents from the time of the Briggs Report onwards gave warnings of trouble ahead unless all interests were catered for. And ''How was it'', they will ask, ''that the Bill was presented as 'Uncontroversial' when two out of the six existing Statutory Bodies had made clear their objections?''.

Behind these and other presenting problems, will they conclude that as far as Health Visitors were concerned, the work of the Council, which in its own estimation was successful, might have contributed perhaps unconsciously to the unsympathetic treatment it received? Firstly, the Council had shown that education and training could take place successfully if based outside the Health Service, which in turn took away a measure of power from Health Departments and from the administrators of the services. This was a break with tradition and the removal of powers is liable to be resisted by Government Departments and by individuals. Secondly, Health Visitors themselves, as a result of a wider form of education, were prepared to question and, on occasions, challenge the views of some others who were trained themselves in isolation for a profession renowned for its hierarchical structure and some of whose leaders were still expecting others to accept their views as necessarily right. In other words, while all might be acting with the best of intentions, their ways of arriving at an answer could be different. Thirdly, the Council had proved that a system of education and training could be conducted on a U.K. basis. While it might have been supposed that this would be an advantage, or even "the shape of things to come" in an Act which was related to the United Kingdom as a whole, this did not fit in with the strong nationalist feelings which had been aroused. Again, traditionally, courses for Nurses and Midwives had been arranged (except for the link between England and Wales) on a national basis, and, indeed, the service itself was in the hands of separate Health Departments which themselves might have different policies. Was the provision of courses within Institutes of Higher and Further Education, the practice of debating issues and the planning on a UK basis wrong in itself, or was it simply out of tune with the thinking of others at that time?

There can be little doubt that the 1979 Act placed the education and training of Health Visitors in a perilous position. At worst, if all decisions by the Central Council and National Boards and the Health Departments took as their focus institutional care alone and Nurses, by reason of superior numbers, carried every vote; if the Chairmen and Chief Officers appointed saw Health Visiting as an unnecessary service or at most as an adjunct to nursing per se in the same category as an individual JBCNS course; if the skilled professional staff of the Council were dispersed to serve the National Boards without regard to retaining a nucleus of expertise to deal with Health Visitor education and training; if courses were taken back into isolation in the Health Service simply to augment Schools of Nursing and Midwifery; if Health Visitors were denied the right to select HVT students and altogether it was assumed Nurses who were not Health Visitors could speak for Health Visitors (but not Health Visitors who were Registered Nurses for Nurses), Health Visitor education and training as it was known could not be maintained. Rather than allow a slow process of decline, it would be kinder if it were announced that Health Visiting was to be phased out and plan accordingly. But, of course, Parliament might have had something to say about that.

But will they "that look back" have seen that at this stage there could be hope? Once the 1979 Act was on the Statute Book all parties declared the intention to leave the disputes of the past behind and to endeavour to make the Act work. This in itself would be no easy task with so many basic matters set aside rather than delay, or possibly halt, the preparations for the Bill to which the Government Department staff were clearly committed. It would be difficult, too, to avoid resurrecting some of the controversial issues when the practical applications of the wording of the Act came under closer scrutiny. Again there would be a great danger then of the staff and the Government Departments rather than the appointed (or elected) members controlling events in line with their own views, especially in the initial stages of uncertainty if disagreement occurs.

Perhaps, however, those that come after will find that a new generation had learnt from the mistakes, mishandlings and misjudgements of the past and was prepared now to listen to others and accommodate different viewpoints, provide for specialist skills on educational grounds and was prepared to challenge ideas and in turn be challenged themselves in open debate without rancour. For then and only then can members of these professions be appreciated by doctors, teachers and civil servants alike and accepted to take their place on equal terms. Then and only then can the talents undoubtedly present within the ranks of Nurses, Midwives and Health Visitors alike be used not only for the benefit of the three professions separately and collectively but also most valuably in the wider world.

And so in the last analysis, how will the efforts of this generation be seen, what were its failures and what were its successes and to what extent if any will this page of history be a source of inspiration? All this, including the part played by the CETHV in the short lifetime it was to be allowed to enjoy, must now be left to the verdict of those who come after.

Footnote: Quotation Dorothy Hall, formerly Regional Officer for Nursing at WHO in Copenhagen in an interview with Alison Dunn - see Nursing Times, June 4 1981. With reference to her posting in SE Asia where she was responsible for nursing projects in ten countries of the region, she said, *"We had a lot of British nurses working in the field and it was there I developed my respect for the British Health Visitor. I saw her doing superb public health nursing - just the kind of care the community needed."*

APPENDIX I

THE COUNCIL 1974-1977

CHAIRMEN:

Dr. Clifford Butler from 1 January 1977	Vice Chancellor	Loughborough University
Sir John Butterfield 1 October 1974 to 31 December 1977.	Regius Professor of Physic	University of Cambridge

MEMBERS:

Mrs. P.M. Boaden	Health Visitor Tutor	Polytechnic of the South Bank
Mrs. J. Brownlie	Councillor	Appointed by Convention of Scottish Local Authorities.
Miss Y.E. Buckoke	Area Nursing Officer	Northumberland AHA
Miss J. Challinor	Head of Department	Sheffield Polytechnic.
Mrs. M.F. Cordon	Health Visitor	Clinic Centre, Greasby, Merseyside.
Miss K.N. Davies	Area Nurse (Child Health)	Coventry AHA
Miss C.M. Fraser	Head of Department	Queen Margaret Coll., Edinburgh
Dr. W.G. Harding	Area Medical Officer	Camden AHA
Mr. R. Hedley	Director	Trent Polytechnic, Nottingham.
Miss M. Illing	Head of Department of Applied Social Studies	Croydon Technical College.
Professor W.G. Irwin	Department of General Practice	Queen's University, Belfast.
Mrs. M. Klinger	Senior HV Tutor	Milton Keynes Coll. of Education
Mrs. R.M. Latham	Borough Councillor	Romford, Essex.
Miss E.M. Llewellyn	Principal Lecturer	W.London Institute
Mr. M.J. McAllister	Vice-Principal	Blackpool College of Technology & Art.
Professor J.K.M. McFarlane	Department of Nursing	Manchester University.
Miss A.W. Maxwell	Health Visitor Tutor	Dundee College of Technology

Miss P. Morton	Area Nursing Officer	Lincolnshire AHA
Dr. M. Murchison	Community Medicine Specialist	Highland Health Board
Miss M. Nairn	Chief Area Nursing Officer	Glasgow Health Board
Mr. V. Pereira-Mendoza	Director	Polytechnic of the South Bank
Dr. A. Reeves	General Practitioner	Normanton, W. Yorks.
Dr. C.J. Revington (resigned July 1976)	Area Medical Officer	Mid Glamorgan AHA
Professor I.M. Richardson	Dept. of General Practice	University of Aberdeen.
Mrs. E.H. Simmonds	Organising Tutor (Retired)	London Boroughs Training Committee.
Miss W.M. Tagg	District Nursing Officer	Clwyd Health Authority.
Miss M. Walton	Area Nursing Officer	Leeds AHA
Miss E.M.K. Welsh	Director of Nursing and Midwifery Education	Northern Ireland Council for Nurses and Midwives
Mrs. M. White	HV/Nursing Officer	Croydon AHA
Mr. S.E. Williams	County Councillor	Avon County
Professor W.M. Williams (appointed July 1976)	Head of Dept. of Sociology	University College of Swansea.

Assessors from DHSS, DES and the appropriate Scottish, Northern Irish and Welsh Government Departments attended all Council meetings, Extraordinary Council meetings and National Advisory Committees as observers.

APPENDIX II

THE COUNCIL 1977-1980

CHAIRMAN:

Dr. Clifford Butler	Vice-Chancellor	Loughborough University

MEMBERS:

Miss H.J. Ash	Senior Lecturer Health Visiting	Gloucestershire Institute of Higher Education
Mrs. G. Barnes	Principal Health Visitor Tutor	North East Surrey College of Technology
Miss B.J. Brown	Health Visitor/ Fieldwork Teacher	Sandwell H.A.
Mrs. J. Brownlie	Councillor	Appointed by Convention of Scottish Local Authorities
Miss J. Challinor	Head of Department	Sheffield Polytechnic
Miss V.A. Chapman	Senior Lecturer	Polytechnic of the South Bank
Miss K.N. Davies	Area Nurse/ Child Health	Coventry A.H.A.
Miss C.M. Fraser	Head of Department	Queen Margaret College Edinburgh
Miss M. Fraser	Principal Lecturer Health Studies	Brighton Polytechnic
Miss W. Frost	Area Nursing Officer	Bedfordshire A.H.A.
Miss M. Illing	Head of Department	Croydon College of Design & Technology
Miss G. Jackson	Director of Training	London Boroughs Training Committee
Mrs. R.M. Latham	Councillor	Romford, Essex
Miss C.M. Lee	Principal Lecturer	Newcastle-upon-Tyne Polytechnic (CNC representative)
Miss M.E. Lindars	Area Nursing Officer	Buckinghamshire A.H.A.
Mrs. L.H. Lipson	Councillor	Appointed by the Association of Metropolitan Authorities
Mr. M.J. McAllister	Principal	Blackpool College of Technology & Art
Miss M.H. McHattie	Div. Nursing Officer	Tayside Health Board

Miss P.M. Matthews	Area Nursing Officer	Dyfed Health Authority
Miss M. Nairn	Chief Area Nursing Officer	Glasgow Health Board
Dr. J.S. Noble	General Practitioner	Ashington, Northumberland
Prof. I.M. Richardson	Professor of General Practice	Aberdeen University
Dr. J.F. Richardson	Principal	Medway & Maidstone College of Technology
Miss M. Watson	Area Nursing Officer	Leeds A.H.A.
Miss E.M. Welsh	Director of Nursing	Northern Ireland Council for Nurses and Midwives
Dr. O.M. White	Pro-Rector	Northern Ireland Polytechnic
Dr. D. Wild	Area Medical Officer	West Sussex A.H.A.
Cllr. S.E. Williams	Chairman	Avon County Social Services Committee
Prof. W.M. Williams	Professor of Sociology and Anthropology	University College Swansea
Mrs. C.T. Wilson	Principal Lecturer in Social Policy	North East London Polytechnic
Dr. T.S. Wilson	Community Medicine Specialist	The Greater Glasgow Health Board

APPENDIX III

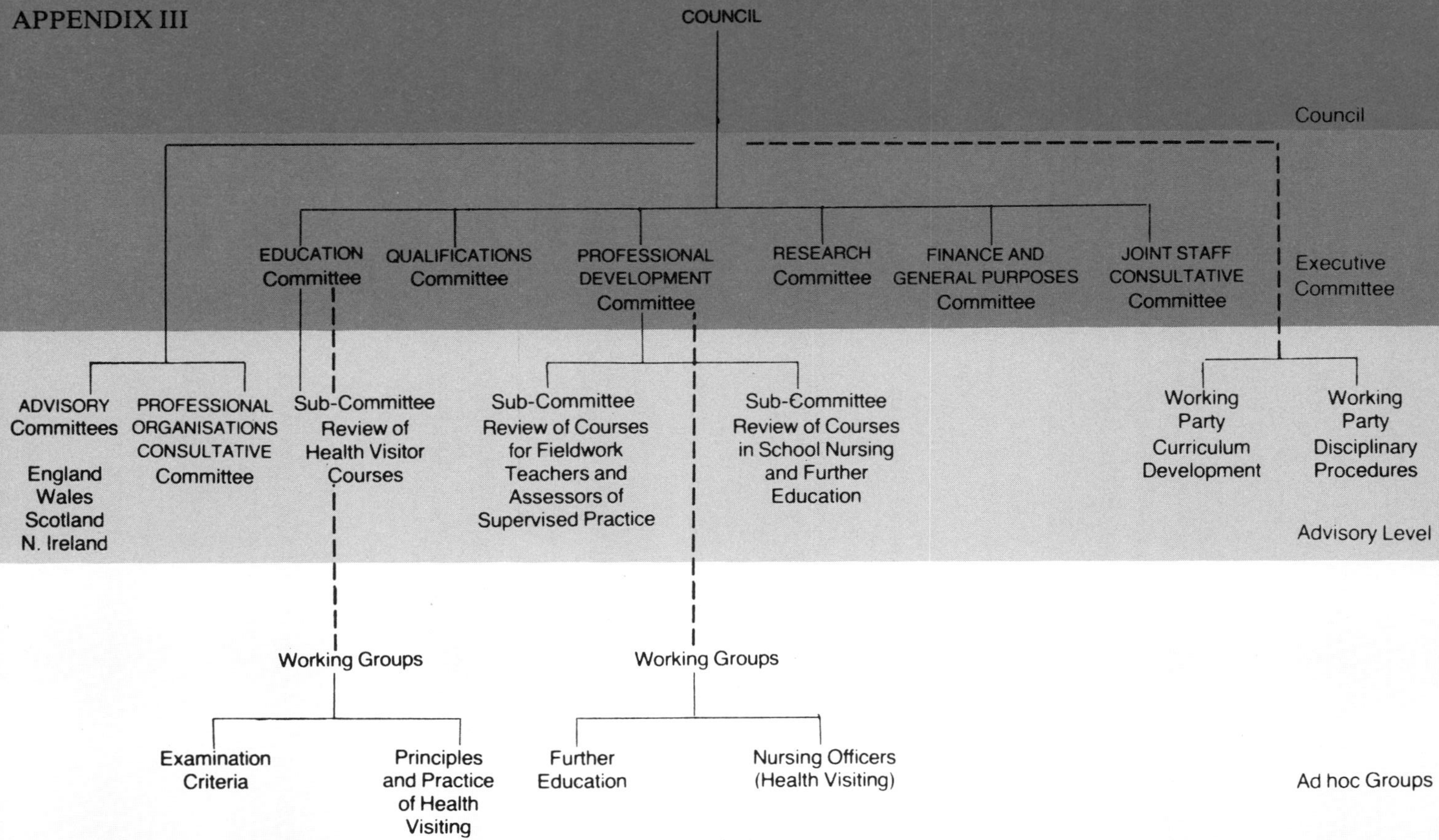

APPENDIX IV

STUDENT NUMBERS

A. *NUMBER OF STUDENTS ENTERING HEALTH VISITOR TRAINING 1975/76 - 1980/81*

Distribution of Post-Registration students by country in which trained.

(One Year Full Time PR)	1975/76	1976/77	1977/78	1978/79	1979/80	1980/81
England	1086	1027	977	1054	1021	969
Scotland	208	178	158	196	184	155
Wales	53	64	56	61	62	55
Northern Ireland	39	37	45	43	41	52
United Kingdom	**1386**	**1306**	**1236**	**1354**	**1308**	**1231**

Number of Students on other courses (all in England, except "Special" in Scotland

Two Year Part Time PR	35	49	21	31	24	35
Combined HV/DN	2	4	3	2	0	0
Degree (includes Manchester University)	43	38	40	22	32	29
Integrated	64	35	16	16	9	0
Modified	6	7	10	9	14	14
Special	5	2	-	-	-	-
TOTAL 1973-4 1974-75	**155**	**135**	**90**	**80**	**79**	**78**

B. *NUMBER OF STUDENTS SUCCESSFULLY COMPLETING HEALTH VISITOR TRAINING 1975/80*

Distribution of students successfully completing Post Registration courses by country in which trained.

(One Year Full Time PR)	1975	1976	1977	1978	1979	1980
England	859	1060	971	940	1010	971
Scotland	141	194	173	157	192	178
Wales	50	46	58	52	58	61
Northern Ireland	37	37	35	44	42	41
United Kingdom	**1087**	**1337**	**1237**	**1193**	**1392**	**1251**

Number of students completing other courses (all in England, except "Special" in Scotland).

Two Year Part Time PR	6	17	32	42	22	31
Combined HV/DN	7	2	4	3	2	-
Degree	17	23	26	27	40	29
Integrated	51	55	41	49	52	39
Modified	3	6	7	10	9	12
Special	-	-	5	2	-	-
TOTAL	**84**	**103**	**115**	**133**	**125**	**111**

C. *FIELDWORK TEACHER COURSE*

(a) *Fieldwork Teacher Part 1 Courses - Letters of Attendance/Statements of Authority*

Year (Jan-Dec)	1975	1976	1977	1978	1979	1980
Letters/Statements issued	314	375	379	330	339	308

4162 Letters/Statements had been issued in toto as at 31 december 1980.

(b) *Fieldwork Teacher Certificates*

Year (Jan-Dec)	1978	1979	1980
No. of certificates issued	920	282	296

D. *HEALTH VISITOR TUTORS*

(a) *No. of HV Tutors entered on Roll*

Year (Jan-Dec)	1975	1976	1977	1978	1979	1980
No. of HV Tutors entered on Roll	42	34	24	34	24	23

(b) 382 names appeared on the Health Visitor Tutor Roll as at 31 December 1980.

E. *REFRESHER COURSES*

Year (Jan-Dec)	1975	1976	1977	1978	1979	1980
No. of HVs attending	965	880	647	458	733	575

F. *SCHOOL NURSES*

Since 15 April 1981 (Council Meeting) the following School Nurses are eligible to receive a Statement of Successful Completion of an Approved Course in School Nursing.

Year (Jan-Dec)	1978	1979	1980
No. of School Nurses	11	75	117

Index